Understanding

HEART
FAILURE

Professor John Cleland

Published by Family Doctor Publications Limited
in association with the British Medical Association

IMPORTANT NOTICE

This book is intended not as a substitute for personal medical advice but as a supplement to that advice for the patient who wishes to understand more about his or her condition.

Before taking any form of treatment YOU SHOULD ALWAYS CONSULT YOUR MEDICAL PRACTITIONER.

In particular (without limit) you should note that advances in medical science occur rapidly and some of the information about drugs and treatment contained in this booklet may very soon be out of date.

© Family Doctor Publications 1998–2002
Updated 1999, 2000, 2002
Second edition 2001

Family Doctor Publications, PO Box 4664, Poole, Dorset BH15 1NN

Medical Editor: Dr Tony Smith
Cover Artist: Dave Eastbury
Medical Artist: Philip Wilson
Design: MPG Design, Blandford Forum, Dorset
Printing: Reflex Litho, Thetford, using acid-free paper

ISBN: 1 898205 78 7

Contents

What is heart failure? 1

How your heart works 5

What causes heart failure? 12

Diagnosing heart failure 22

The right treatment 33

How to help yourself 49

Living with heart failure 56

New frontiers 68

Useful addresses 71

Index 75

What is heart failure?

CASE HISTORY: ERIC

Eric was 67 when he was taken to hospital with severe pains in the middle of his chest. Tests showed that he'd had a heart attack. He recovered without any further problems but felt exhausted most of the time. In the following months he noticed he was gaining weight and getting more and more breathless, even walking at a gentle pace. Three months after his heart attack, he found he could no longer walk even to the newsagents without stopping to catch his breath. Eric went to see his GP, who examined him. His GP suspected that he might have heart failure, took a blood test (to check for anaemia or a kidney problem), organised a special test at the local hospital (an echocardiogram) and gave him some water tablets. Over the next few days Eric passed a lot more urine, lost four to five pounds (two to two and a half kilograms) in weight and his breathlessness greatly improved. The hospital test confirmed that he had developed heart failure as a result of the heart attack and indicated that further treatment could help to keep the problem under control.

HEART FAILURE

- Means that the heart can no longer do its work properly without some medical help
- With medical help symptoms may be controlled and reasonable quality of life maintained for many years
- About 100,000 people develop heart failure in the UK each year

WHAT IS HEART FAILURE?

Heart failure sounds frightening, but doctors actually use the term to describe all the situations where the heart cannot keep up with the demands made on it by the body; the heart fails to do its job, which is to pump enough blood around the body. This may cause symptoms. With medical help, usually pills/tablets, the heart can generally manage well enough.

When a doctor says someone is suffering from heart failure, the family's natural reaction is to assume the worst.

Heart failure can be the end-result of many heart problems, so it is important to find out why it has happened. The most common cause is coronary artery disease. This is a condition in which the blood vessels that supply oxygen and nutrients to the heart muscle become partly or completely blocked. A heart that is starved of an adequate blood supply will fail to work normally.

Heart failure can also develop in people who have had high blood pressure for a long time.

There are many other rarer causes of heart failure, some needing different treatments, so it is important for your doctor to find out the cause in your particular case.

In most cases, medication can help to strengthen the action of the heart and relieve the symptoms of heart failure.

SYMPTOM GUIDE

A person with heart failure may have one or more of the following symptoms, but other medical problems can also cause similar symptoms:

- shortness of breath which gets worse during exercise or with lying flat
- needing to sleep sitting up or waking at night with severe breathlessness
- coughing and/or wheezing especially at night
- swollen ankles and weight gain caused by fluid retention
- unexplained weight loss
- tiredness

Symptoms

The main ones are breathlessness, swollen ankles and tiredness, but there can be many other reasons for this combination of symptoms and your doctor must make the diagnosis. How severe the symptoms are depends on the amount of damage done to the heart. The main symptoms are listed briefly in the box below, but we will look at symptoms in detail in the chapter starting on page 22. However, it is important to remember that no two people are likely to have exactly the same combination of symptoms and some will have more problems than others.

Who gets heart failure?

Heart failure is uncommon in people under the age of 50, but it affects progressively more people in older age groups. The principal cause of heart failure between the ages of 50 and 75 is a heart attack. In a heart attack one of the blood vessels taking oxygen to the heart muscle becomes blocked. As a result part of the heart muscle dies. So anything that makes a heart attack more likely also increases the risk of heart failure. This means that people who smoke, have high blood pressure or high blood cholesterol or who have diabetes are more likely to develop heart failure.

It is also possible for heart failure to occur without being preceded by a heart attack. High blood pressure is sometimes an important cause. Narrowed or leaking heart valves may cause heart failure in people of any age but are also more common in older people. Occasionally, drinking excessive amounts of alcohol can poison the heart muscle. Abstinence from alcohol may allow a partial or even full recovery.

Rarer causes of heart failure may affect pregnant women and people with muscular dystrophy and, more rarely still, children and unborn babies can experience heart failure.

Case history: Ken

Ken, a widower aged 75, had been well until he started having problems getting about because of his shortness of breath. He found he could no longer climb stairs or hurry for the bus without getting out of breath. He went to his GP, who told him that there was some fluid on his lungs and prescribed water tablets (diuretics) to clear it. Before long, Ken was feeling much more like his old self. An echocardiography test (see page 29) at the local hospital showed a narrowed (aortic) valve. Three months after valve replacement he is back to normal.

Case history: Lily

Lily, an 81-year-old woman, was brought by her daughter to see her

GP because she was worried that her mother seemed to be getting very tired, with swollen ankles, breathlessness and was becoming confused at night.

She had enjoyed good health until recently apart from long-standing (15 years) high blood pressure, for which she had been given treatment, although she often forgot to take it. The doctor suggested that heart failure resulting from the high blood pressure might be the cause of all her problems, including the confusion. He arranged for an echocardiography test at the local hospital which showed that the heart had indeed been damaged by the high blood pressure. Treatment with water pills and a medicine called an angiotensin-converting enzyme (ACE) inhibitor rapidly improved her symptoms, including her confusion.

CASE HISTORY: IRENE

Irene had a heart attack two years ago, and for the last few months she'd been having symptoms that gradually got worse. Her ankles were often very swollen and she was short of breath, and recently she'd started waking in the night unable to get her breath. Her GP arranged for her to see the specialist at hospital outpatients. Tests confirmed heart failure. The patient responded well to a combination of medicines, including a beta-blocker, ACE inhibitor and 'water pill'.

KEY POINTS

✓ Heart attacks and high blood pressure are the most common reasons for people to develop heart failure

✓ There are highly effective treatments for heart failure

How your heart works

Together, the heart and all the blood vessels around the body form what's called the cardiovascular system.

Your heart is actually a pump made of muscle. The heart is made from a special type of muscle not found anywhere else in the body, so it doesn't get tired the way ordinary muscles do. Its task is to keep your body supplied with the nutrients and oxygen that are dissolved in your blood. The arteries carry the blood away from the heart and the veins bring it back; the direction of blood flow through the heart is controlled by valves which open to let blood through, then close tightly to prevent it going back the wrong way.

In order to do its job properly, your heart muscle must be working normally – it can't pump efficiently if it is damaged. Damage can be to a part of the muscle, for example, an area of dead heart muscle from

a heart attack is eventually replaced by a scar that doesn't contract when the rest of the muscle does. Damage can also be widespread involving all of the heart muscle, as happens in dilated cardiomyopathy (see page 20). In these cases the individual muscle fibres can't function properly. The heart also has to beat regularly at an appropriate rate, depending on what activity you're involved in at any given time. The valves that control the flow of blood must also be in good condition to keep blood flowing in the right direction.

The heart is divided into separate halves which beat together but pump blood to different parts of the body. The right side receives 'used' blood from the body and sends it off to the lungs to be replenished with oxygen. The left side receives the oxygenated blood from the lungs and pumps it around the body. Each side of the

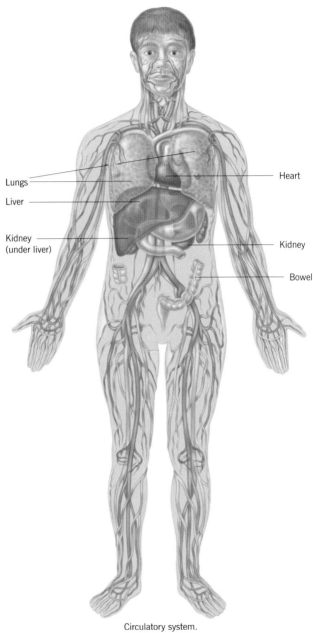

Lungs

Liver

Kidney
(under liver)

Heart

Kidney

Bowel

Circulatory system.

heart has an upper and lower chamber. The upper ones, called the atria, are where blood is collected from the veins. When valves leading to the lower chambers (the ventricles) open, the atria contract, emptying the blood into the ventricles. Those valves close and the exit valves into the arteries open. The ventricles then contract in their turn, and the blood is pumped out into the arteries. The contractions of both the upper and lower chambers of the heart are controlled by a network of special electrical tissue throughout the heart. An area in the atria acts as a pacemaker, ensuring that the heart beats regularly and evenly.

If the heart rhythm becomes irregular (as in atrial fibrillation, see page 16), the chambers may not have time to fill properly or empty completely, so reducing the amount of blood being pumped out. Similarly, if the heart is beating too fast or too slowly (see Palpitations, page 54), it can't work efficiently.

The average person has about five litres (eight pints) of blood, which circulates right round the body in one minute while you're at rest. When you exert yourself physically, your heart speeds up and pumps harder, and may pump as much as 25 or 30 litres in a minute. A failing heart is not capable of doing this, which is why vigorous exercise of any kind becomes difficult.

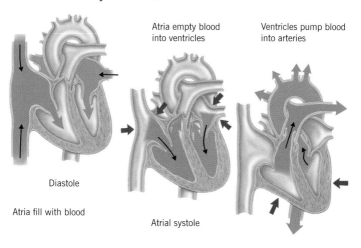

Atria empty blood into ventricles

Ventricles pump blood into arteries

Diastole

Atria fill with blood

Atrial systole

Ventricular systole

Heart pumping cycle.

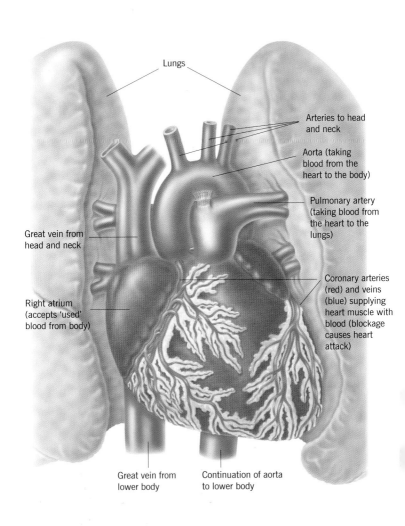

Lungs

Arteries to head and neck

Aorta (taking blood from the heart to the body)

Pulmonary artery (taking blood from the heart to the lungs)

Great vein from head and neck

Coronary arteries (red) and veins (blue) supplying heart muscle with blood (blockage causes heart attack)

Right atrium (accepts 'used' blood from body)

Great vein from lower body

Continuation of aorta to lower body

The heart and great vessels.

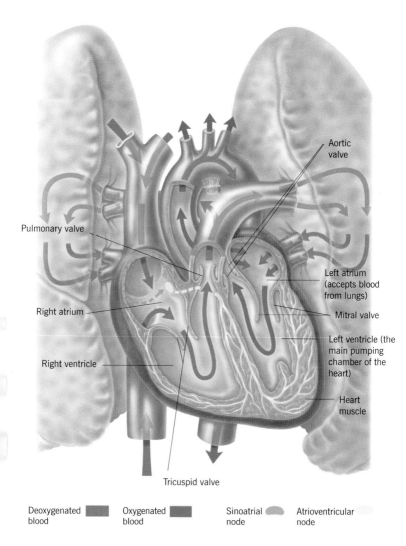

Aortic
valve

Pulmonary valve

Right atrium

Right ventricle

Left atrium
(accepts blood
from lungs)

Mitral valve

Left ventricle (the
main pumping
chamber of the
heart)

Heart
muscle

Tricuspid valve

Deoxygenated
blood

Oxygenated
blood

Sinoatrial
node

Atrioventricular
node

Internal anatomy of the heart. Arrows indicate direction of blood flow.

WHEN THE HEART STARTS TO FAIL . . .

Blood continues to return to the heart but if it is not working efficiently the heart may not be able to keep up. The pressure backs up into the circulation too. As a result the tiny blood vessels known as capillaries begin to leak fluid into the tissues. This can happen in the lungs or elsewhere in the body, causing **swelling**. This is most obvious in the ankles where fluid collects under the influence of gravity.

As there is less blood reaching the kidneys they can't work as efficiently either. They pass out less salt and water than usual and even more fluid collects in the tissues.

When fluid leaks into the lungs it takes up space which should have been filled with air, reducing the amount of oxygen reaching the blood, and so the person becomes **short of breath**. They may feel **tired** because their muscles are not getting all the oxygen and nutrients they require and waste products are accumulating rather than being carried away in the bloodstream as they should be. We will look more closely at the symptoms of heart failure on page 22.

Recent research has identified a variety of hormones (chemical messengers) and nerves that send signals from a failing heart to change the way the kidneys and blood vessels work. Some of these changes help to relieve the load on the heart; others increase it.

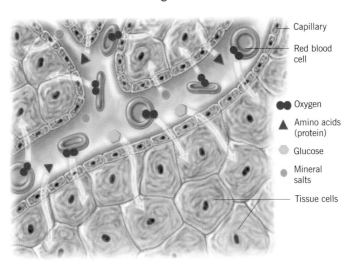

Capillary

Red blood cell

Oxygen

Amino acids (protein)

Glucose

Mineral salts

Tissue cells

Blood supplying tissues with nutrients and oxygen.

There are many different types of medications for treating heart failure and, as they work in different ways, they can often be combined. Some work by correcting or controlling the underlying problem, some control symptoms and some do both. We will look at how some of these medicines work on page 33.

KEY POINTS

✓ Your heart is a pump made of muscle

✓ The average person has about five litres of blood circulating round the body in one minute when at rest

✓ A failing heart cannot pump harder which is why vigorous exercise is difficult

What causes heart failure?

There are many reasons why heart failure can occur. Which is most likely depends on the age of the individual concerned.

HEART ATTACK

In a heart attack, one or more of the blood vessels taking oxygen to the heart muscle become blocked. As a result part of the heart muscle dies. A heart attack is also known as a 'coronary' or a 'myocardial infarction'. It is the most common cause of heart failure in people between the ages of 50 and 75 years. A heart attack usually happens because of a complete blockage in one or more of the blood vessels that supply the heart muscle itself with oxygen. These are known as the coronary arteries and, over a number of years, they can become narrowed because of what is known as atheroma. Atheroma means that fatty deposits called plaques are laid down on the lining of the coronary arteries, gradually reducing the space through which blood can flow. Eventually, these plaques can split. When this happens, a blood clot (or thrombosis) forms over the damaged area and completely blocks the artery. The blood clot

RISK FACTORS FOR A HEART ATTACK

- Smoking
- High blood pressure
- High cholesterol levels
- Generally unhealthy lifestyle (stress, diet, exercise, obesity)

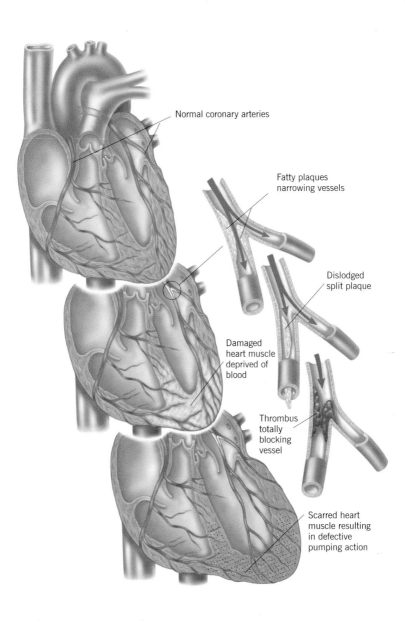

Normal coronary arteries

Fatty plaques narrowing vessels

Dislodged split plaque

Damaged heart muscle deprived of blood

Thrombus totally blocking vessel

Scarred heart muscle resulting in defective pumping action

Atheroma may block the coronary arteries and cause a heart attack.

forms as the damaged tissues release chemicals which activate the clotting system. This is why the so-called 'clot-busting' medicines are often used to treat heart attacks.

When an artery is blocked in this way, part of the heart muscle is starved of blood and dies. Over the next few weeks, this damaged area is replaced by scar tissue which cannot contract with the rest of the muscle when the heart beats. This interferes with the efficient working of the heart and may lead to heart failure. Prompt hospital treatment with appropriate medicines (see page 33) can, if given in the first few hours after the attack, reduce the amount of damage done and improve the healing process. The amount of muscle that is damaged in large part determines whether the person will develop heart failure. Occasionally, a heart attack can damage the muscle that supports a heart valve, causing the valve to leak. This can also lead to heart failure.

Roughly one person in every three who has a heart attack will show some evidence of heart failure. In some people, it may be mild and perhaps temporary. Around one in five of those who do not have any problems initially will go on to develop heart failure in the next 5–10 years, although treatment may prevent or at least delay it. Unfortunately, in some people damage to the heart muscle is so extensive that severe heart failure develops rapidly and may be difficult to control.

HIGH BLOOD PRESSURE

Blood pressure actually means the pressure in the arteries. With each beat of the heart, it rises to a high point (systolic pressure), then falls to its lowest point between beats (diastolic pressure). Both are measured using a device called a sphygmomanometer and recorded as millimetres of mercury (or mmHg). Most people will have had this test done at some time (see page 26).

As the cuff around your arm is inflated, it eventually tightens sufficiently to stop the blood flow in the lower arm for a few seconds. The air is then let out, gradually lowering the pressure, while the doctor, nurse or machine itself listens to the artery at the elbow for the sounds made by the blood as the flow returns to normal. The two pressures – systolic and diastolic – are usually expressed as, for example, 170/90 or 170 over 90. A healthy person's blood pressure should be around 120/70; in the older population 140/90 is a borderline increase and 150/100 is definitely raised.

Most people with high blood pressure have what is known as

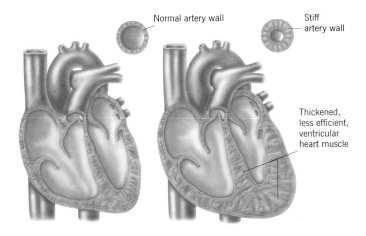

Normal artery wall

Stiff artery wall

Thickened, less efficient, ventricular heart muscle

Normal heart and vessels.

Heart and vessels damaged by high blood pressure.

'essential hypertension' – that is, their blood pressure is raised for no apparent reason. The triggering factors for essential hypertension are unclear, but obesity, high salt intake and high cholesterol may play a role. Less commonly high blood pressure is caused by kidney disease or diseases of other glands.

Someone with high blood pressure will probably have no symptoms at all, which is why it is important to have regular checks. If your blood pressure is found to be raised, your doctor will probably repeat the test several times over the next few weeks and, if it stays high, you'll be put on long-term medication to bring it down. You must keep taking the tablets, even though you have no symptoms and can't feel any benefit; unless your

blood pressure is kept under control, it could eventually damage your heart and it also increases the risk of a stroke.

The higher the pressure, the harder the heart has to work. Not only is raised pressure a common cause of heart attacks, it may also cause heart failure in older people who have never actually had a heart attack and even occasionally in younger people if it is high enough.

With prolonged high blood pressure the heart muscle gets thicker and more bulky as it continues to try to pump blood around the body. This thickened muscle is stiffer and actually functions less well than normal heart muscle. High pressure also damages the walls of the arteries over time. They become stiffer, and this in turn raises the pressure in the system further, increasing the risk of a heart attack or stroke. All this takes place gradually over a period of years, so the earlier high blood pressure is treated, the better the chances of delaying or even preventing the onset of heart failure or other complications of high blood pressure. Even when heart failure has already developed, it's important to treat high blood pressure, because this makes it easier for the heart to pump efficiently.

ATRIAL FIBRILLATION

In this condition, the upper chambers of the heart (the atria) beat at a much faster rate than they should. The lower chambers (the ventricles) also beat fast and irregularly, reducing the pumping efficiency of the heart and often causing heart failure. There are many possible reasons why atrial fibrillation may occur, but the most common is coronary artery disease or sometimes a heart attack. About a quarter of cases of heart failure are caused or complicated by atrial fibrillation. For many people, treatment with medicines can restore a normal heart rhythm. Some people may be admitted to hospital for the day to have their heart rhythm

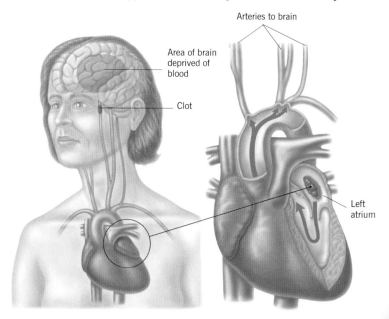

Arteries to brain

Area of brain deprived of blood

Clot

Left atrium

Clot forming in the atria then causing a stroke.

converted back to normal by an electric shock. This is generally performed under a general anaesthetic.

Even when it's not possible to return the heart rhythm to normal, medicines can be prescribed to slow the rate down and so allow the heart to pump more efficiently.

A further problem with atrial fibrillation is that pools of relatively stagnant blood form in the atria which are not emptying completely. Clots form in blood that is stagnant anywhere in the body, so clots can form in the atria.

A small piece of clot may break off and be released into the circulation. If a clot becomes lodged in a blood vessel in the brain, it can cause a stroke – meaning an area of brain tissue dies from lack of oxygen. Most commonly this causes paralysis or weakness in an arm and/or leg. Clots can also cause problems elsewhere, for example, if a blood vessel in the leg is blocked. If the clot is in a major artery, the leg will become very painful as it has lost its blood supply. Untreated, gangrene can develop. To prevent these sorts of problems, people with atrial fibrillation often need to take tablets (such as warfarin) to reduce blood clotting or 'thin the blood'.

VALVE DISEASE

The purpose of a heart valve is to allow blood to flow in one direction only. This means that it will let blood into a chamber or major vessel, but won't let it back out the way it came in.

There are two ways in which a heart valve can become damaged:

- It can become narrowed (stenosis), so not enough blood can be pushed through the gap with each beat of the heart; the heart tries to pump harder, putting it under extra strain.

- It can become leaky or incompetent (regurgitation). In this case, some blood will flow back into the chamber that it came from, so again the heart needs to work harder to pump enough blood out in the right direction.

Any of the four heart valves may become diseased, but the mitral or aortic valves are most often affected. This is because they are both in the left side of the heart which is exposed to much higher pressures and stresses than the right side. Over 99 per cent of heart valve operations are on one or other of these valves.

Older people may have suffered damage to their heart valves as a consequence of having had rheumatic fever in childhood or early adult life, but, fortunately, this illness is now rare in the developed world. Valves may also be damaged by infections (such as endocarditis – see box on page 19) or by some immune system disorders. Valves may leak or become stiff simply as part of the ageing process.

The box on page 19 lists the most common causes of valvular heart disease (VHD) in terms of stenosis or regurgitation, although it is quite possible to have 'mixed valve disease', i.e. a combination of the two.

Sometimes you may be aware that you have a problem with a heart valve before you get any symptoms. This is particularly common if you have a congenital (or inborn) defect which has been picked up by chance or in the course of having tests for some other routine operation. Not everyone who has a diseased heart valve will need an operation. Some people can live happily all their life with no symptoms at all, and others may respond well to other treatments such as medicines.

HEART MUSCLE DISEASE

Some people with poorly functioning heart muscles have normal coronary arteries, excluding coronary disease, and the doctor must look elsewhere for the cause of the damage. Sometimes, none can be found; this condition is known as cardiomyopathy. The disease sometimes runs in families, when it has a genetic basis. There is no doubt that drinking

Competent valves

Incompetent valves

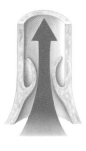

Normal opening

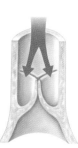

Normal closing

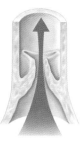

Abnormal opening
– stenosed valve

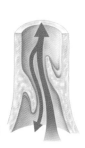

Abnormal closing
– leaking valve

Valve problems.

CAUSES OF VALVE DISEASE

Causes of valvular stenosis	Description
Rheumatic fever	An infection, usually caught in childhood Uncommon to get this nowadays, but people who had it many years ago have now become old enough to have the associated heart problems
Calcification	As we get older many tissues in the body get calcium deposits in them, making them harder and less supple. This happens in the heart valves, but is much faster and more severe in some people than others
Congenital	These are defects that we are born with, and are sometimes inherited from our parents' genes. They may show up immediately after birth, later in life or not at all, depending on their nature and severity

Causes of valvular regurgitation	Description
Rheumatic fever	See above
Ischaemic	After a heart attack, dead areas of heart muscle may involve the cords and tendons that operate the valve, making it leak
Congenital	See above
Floppy valves	Results from degeneration of the valve tissue
Infective (endocarditis)	An infection of a heart valve is extremely serious, and is often a life-threatening emergency
Long-standing high blood pressure	

excessive quantities of alcohol (regular heavy drinking over a number of years) poisons the heart muscle and can cause heart failure. It is also possible for cardiomyopathy to be the result of a virus infection.

In most cases, the heart becomes large and baggy and does not pump very well. Occasionally, the muscle may become thick and stiff instead. When this happens, the person is said to have hypertrophic cardiomyopathy. Although the heart muscle has more bulk, it cannot pump properly.

Overall, heart muscle disease accounts for only about one in fifty of those people with heart failure, but it is responsible for a much higher proportion of cases in young people.

CAN OTHER DISEASES PLAY A PART?

People who already have heart failure or who could be at risk after a heart attack should be checked (and treated if possible) for any other illnesses that might bring on heart failure or make it worse. Anaemia, thyroid and kidney problems are the main causes of concern.

Anaemia

One of the many components that go to make up blood is haemoglobin, which gives it its red colour and holds the oxygen carried in the bloodstream to the tissues. If the red blood cell count is low (anaemia), the blood is less efficient at carrying oxygen, the most essential 'nutrient' for the body.

This means that not only is the heart muscle receiving less oxygen, but it also has to work harder to supply the tissues with all the oxygen that they need. It's easy to see how the additional workload created by the anaemia can put a strain on an already damaged heart and so cause heart failure.

There are many reasons why people develop anaemia, including heavy menstrual periods in women or bleeding in the gut. Sometimes an inadequate diet or a genetic disorder may be responsible. The good news is that, although anaemia is quite common, it is usually easily treated.

Thyroid problems

The thyroid gland produces a hormone which regulates the rate at which most of the body's functions work, including the heart. An over- or under-active gland can cause problems. Anyone who has developed atrial fibrillation should always have a blood test to check whether their thyroid is functioning normally.

Kidney problems

The heart and kidneys work closely together, so when one runs into problems it is bound to affect the other. The kidneys are responsible for getting rid of excess water and salt from the body and, when they stop working properly, too much of both of these is retained. Fluid retention will cause weight gain. Clothing or rings may become tighter and the person may develop symptoms such as breathlessness and ankle swelling – which are similar to those caused by heart failure. What's more, having too much fluid in your circulation can put an added strain on the heart.

On the other hand, heart failure means less blood reaches the kidneys, reducing their efficiency so they can't get rid of fluid properly. In turn, this can make heart failure worse. Kidney problems can be excluded by a simple blood test.

THE DIFFERENCE BETWEEN HEART DISEASE AND HEART FAILURE

Just because you have a problem with your heart, it doesn't mean that you are bound to develop heart failure. For example, most people who have angina don't have heart failure. Their main problem is chest pain which usually comes on when they exercise and stops when they rest. It is caused by reduced blood flow to the heart muscle itself.

The term 'heart failure' only tells you that the heart is not working well enough to pump nutrients and oxygen to the tissues – it doesn't tell you why. In fact, as we have seen, there are several possible explanations.

KEY POINTS

✓ Heart failure has many causes

✓ Different causes of heart disease may require different treatment

---

Diagnosing heart failure

SPOTTING THE SYMPTOMS

Having looked at the way the heart and circulation work, it may be easier to understand why heart failure causes the symptoms that it does.

Breathlessness

Usually, this means feeling short of breath when doing some activity that wouldn't normally cause any problems for someone of a similar age – such as walking up a short flight of stairs. In most cases, the breathlessness will have got worse over a period of days, weeks or months. At worst, you may even feel short of breath while resting. However, you must remember that there are many other conditions, such as asthma and chronic bronchitis, that can cause breathlessness, so don't jump to conclusions.

When the problem is caused by heart failure, it can eventually be seriously disabling, so that the person feels breathless even when lying down. One of the features typical of severe heart failure is needing to sleep propped up in bed, sometimes with five or six pillows. You may find that you wake up feeling very short of breath because you have slipped down in the bed. Sitting upright or getting out of bed will usually ease the breathing after 20 minutes or so, but if it doesn't you should phone your doctor who will probably give you an injection of a diuretic to clear the excess fluid quickly. Even if your symptoms do settle fairly promptly, waking at night with severe breathlessness means that your heart failure is not well controlled and you should see your doctor soon.

The reasons why heart failure causes breathlessness are not fully understood, but fluid retention and back pressure from the heart on the lungs make it harder for oxygen to

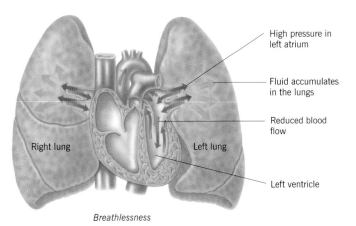

High pressure in
left atrium

Fluid accumulates
in the lungs

Reduced blood
flow

Left ventricle

Right lung

Left lung

Breathlessness

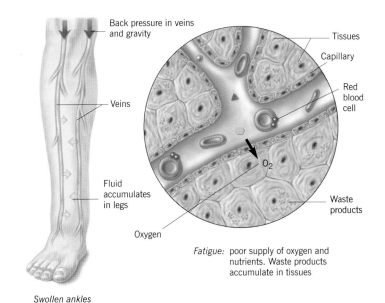

Back pressure in veins
and gravity

Tissues

Capillary

Red
blood
cell

Veins

Fluid
accumulates
in legs

Oxygen

O₂

Waste
products

Fatigue: poor supply of oxygen and
nutrients. Waste products
accumulate in tissues

Swollen ankles

Symptoms of heart failure.

reach the blood. As the heart failure worsens, the small airspaces in the lungs fill up with fluid, making breathing even more difficult.

Swollen ankles

Many normal, healthy people get mildly swollen ankles at times, for example, in hot weather, before a menstrual period or in pregnancy, or if they have varicose veins. However, increasing ankle swelling may be a symptom of heart failure, in which case it is likely to affect both legs equally. In the same way that heart failure causes fluid in the lungs to collect and cause breathlessness, it can also cause fluid to leak out of blood vessels in the body and collect in the tissues, especially the legs.

The actual cause of the leakage is complicated but in simple terms, as the pressure in the heart rises, this causes the pressure in the veins to rise. This creates a back pressure that causes fluid to leak from the blood vessels. Fluid collects most commonly in the ankles simply because of the force of gravity. In worsening heart failure, the swelling can creep further up the legs.

Pressing your thumb into the swollen area for 30 seconds will leave a dent which takes a couple of minutes to disappear. Staying in bed may get rid of swelling round the ankles, but the fluid may collect around the lower part of the back instead.

There are other reasons why one leg suddenly swells up. If the leg is painful, you should see a doctor immediately as this might be the result of a blood clot in one of the leg veins.

Passing more urine at night

As everyone's kidneys work more efficiently when they're lying down, people with heart failure sometimes notice that they pass more urine during the night. Again, there could be other explanations for this – such as an enlarged prostate in men.

Fatigue

This can be a symptom of virtually any medical problem or a normal response to overdoing things. Everyone feels tired at some time but if you're tired all the time without any obvious reason, you should see your doctor. Fatigue can be a symptom of many diseases, including mental stress, depression and viral infections, as well as of heart failure.

A person with heart failure may feel constantly tired because of the poor supply of oxygen and nutrients and the accumulation of waste products in their muscles.

Remember . . .

Heart failure can only be diagnosed

by a doctor after he or she has heard about the symptoms and examined the patient. Generally, some simple tests will also be needed to confirm the diagnosis (see below).

IS IT HEART FAILURE?
How your doctors decide what's wrong

Diagnosing heart failure has to be left to the experts because all the main symptoms can be caused by other illnesses or can sometimes affect normal healthy people. Although, by hearing an account of your symptoms and examining you, the doctor may have enough information to make the diagnosis, most people will also need some tests to confirm it and to find the cause of the heart failure. It is important to detect heart failure as early as possible so that the underlying problem can be put right or at least treated so it doesn't get any worse.

Tests

Your symptoms, together with the physical examination, may be enough for your doctor to say that you are suffering from heart failure. More often than not, however, you'll need to have some tests to confirm the diagnosis and find the cause. A set of guidelines, drawn up by doctors who are experts on the subject, recommends that anyone with suspected heart failure should have the tests shown in the table.

CHECKS AND TESTS

Most people should have the following basic investigations if heart failure is suspected and some may need further more specialised tests afterwards. We look at all these in more detail in the next few pages.

- Physical examination – this is likely to include taking your pulse and blood pressure, listening to your heart, checking the veins in your neck and looking for any swelling
- Blood test
- Chest X-ray
- ECG (electrocardiogram)
- Echocardiogram

PHYSICAL EXAMINATION

Check	What	Why
Pulse	How fast?	A heart that beats too quickly or too slowly cannot pump efficiently
	Is it regular?	Conditions such as atrial fibrillation which cause irregular heartbeat can lead to heart failure
	Character	Sometimes the feel of the pulse can be a clue to problems such as valve disease
Blood pressure	Too high?	High blood pressure can put a strain on the heart and cause heart failure in the long term
	Too low?	This can cause dizziness, blackouts or kidney problems

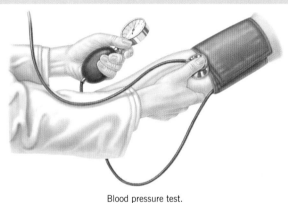

Blood pressure test.

Heart	How it sounds	Any noises heard between the normal sounds of the valves opening and closing indicate turbulent blood flow from a narrowed or leaky valve
Neck	Vein distended?	When the heart isn't pumping properly, pressure backs up in the veins and the vein in the side of the neck becomes distended
Ankles	Swollen?	Fluid can collect in the lower legs and the lower back and occasionally people with heart failure have swollen stomachs

BLOOD TEST

This is to check for anaemia and kidney problems, both of which can make heart failure worse (see pages 20–1). If your heart rhythm is irregular, your blood will also be tested for thyroid hormone levels. An overactive gland can cause atrial fibrillation (see page 16).

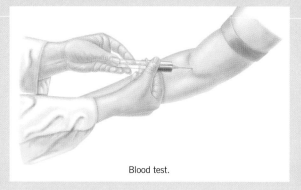

Blood test.

CHEST X-RAY

This simple and familiar test produces a variety of useful information:
- The size and shape of the heart and whether it has changed, by becoming enlarged, for example
- Whether fluid has collected in the airspaces of the lungs as a result of heart failure
- Whether there is any lung disease causing breathlessness.

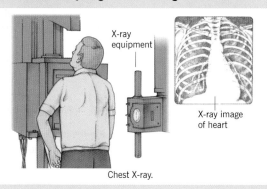

X-ray equipment

X-ray image of heart

Chest X-ray.

ECG (ELECTROCARDIOGRAM)

Every time the heart beats, it causes natural electrical changes, and the ECG records this activity in different sites around the body. The electrical signals are picked up through pads attached across the chest and at other points such as ankles or wrists. These ECG traces give the doctor lots of information about the heart, depending on whether and how they differ from the normal patterns. The doctor can assess heart rate and rhythm and whether the heart muscle is conducting electricity normally. Damaged muscle or muscle that is short of oxygen produces a different tracing.

If the problem is intermittent irregular heartbeats, it can be difficult to spot on a simple ECG tracing when the heart may happen to be beating normally. One way of getting round this situation is for the person to wear a very small portable ECG machine on a belt or over their shoulder for 24 hours. Any time the person feels any symptoms, they press a button which marks the recording. When the results are analysed later, the symptom marker can be compared with the tracing of the heartbeat at that time. Some machines record a heart tracing which can be transmitted down a telephone line to a doctor for an instant opinion or advice.

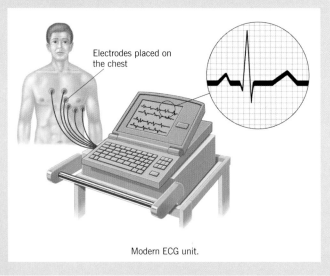

Electrodes placed on the chest

Modern ECG unit.

ECHOCARDIOGRAM

This test involves bouncing sound waves into the heart from a plastic probe placed on the chest. The technique is much the same as the ultrasound scans used to check unborn babies during pregnancy. It allows the doctor to see how the heart muscle and valves are working. This is particularly useful as the doctor can actually see the heart beating and check different areas for problems.

Your own doctor may be able to do the blood test and ECG, but the chest X-ray and echocardiogram usually have to be done at a hospital. Depending on the local set-up, you may or may not have to see a heart specialist. Although specialist services are available in most areas of the country, waiting lists are sometimes long. Many hospitals are setting up special clinics to provide an efficient service for people with heart failure, and echocardiography is becoming more widely available.

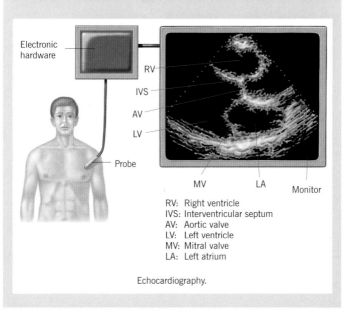

Electronic hardware

RV
IVS
AV
LV

Probe

MV   LA   Monitor

RV: Right ventricle
IVS: Interventricular septum
AV: Aortic valve
LV: Left ventricle
MV: Mitral valve
LA: Left atrium

Echocardiography.

Further investigations

If the results of these tests show that you could benefit from an operation or other special treatment, you might need some extra tests.

EXERCISE TEST

Using a treadmill or bicycle: this helps the specialist to decide how well your heart copes with exercise. Electrodes are placed on your chest and your heart is monitored at varying levels of exercise.

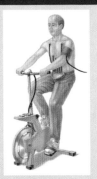

Exercise test using bicycle (right).

HEART SCAN

There are several versions, some of which involve injecting a very small amount of radioactive material into the bloodstream and then using a special camera to measure various aspects of heart function.

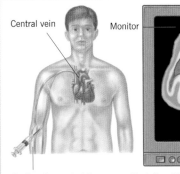

Central vein

Monitor

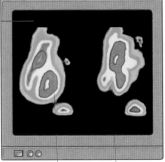

Radioactive material injected into arm vein

The left ventricle is relaxed and filling with blood

The left ventricle is pumping blood out

Heart scan.

ANGIOGRAM

This may be needed if you are having surgery on a valve or a blocked coronary artery. Fine tubes are threaded through blood vessels in your groin or arm under local anaesthetic and threaded up to your heart. Special dye is then injected which allows X-rays to be taken to assess the severity of any problem in the valve or artery and what, if anything, needs to be done to correct it.

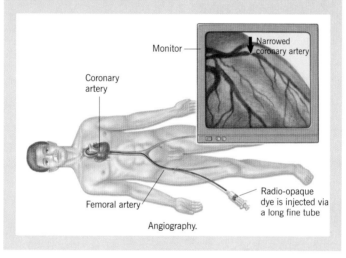

Monitor

Narrowed coronary artery

Coronary artery

Radio-opaque dye is injected via a long fine tube

Femoral artery

Angiography.

KEY POINTS

Most patients require hospital tests to:

✓ Ensure that heart failure is the cause of the symptoms

✓ Discover what the cause of the heart failure is

✓ Discover what other complicating factors there are

The right treatment

When treating heart failure, doctors have simple and clear aims in mind:

- To stop things getting worse for as long as possible in a person who feels well
- To help someone who does not feel well to feel better and enable them to do more
- To prolong the person's life.

What treatment each person has will depend on his or her condition. Most types of treatment that maintain or improve the way the person feels will also help them to live longer. Sometimes, however, treatment that is given to prolong life may have side effects and these may not be acceptable to some people.

MEDICAL TREATMENT

Usually, a person with heart failure will need medical treatment, although some may benefit from surgery as well. As we have seen, heart failure can sometimes be the result of another underlying illness such as thyroid or kidney disease, so the first step is to correct any such problem if at all possible. For some people, this may be all the treatment that is needed. When the main problem is atrial fibrillation (see page 16), the answer may be a treatment called cardioversion which involves giving the heart a brief electric shock (see pages 44 and 47). For most people with heart failure, however, regular, long-term medicines will be needed to help the heart function as near normally as possible.

Medical treatment is a very complex subject with a large number of medicines on the market. The matter is further complicated by the fact that the pharmaceutical companies all give their products 'proprietary/trade' names as well as their actual 'scientific/generic' name. The consequence of this is that, if one medicine is manufactured by three different companies, it will have three different names depending on where you get it from. This can be confusing as you may be on exactly the same medication as somebody you know but you each have different names on the boxes of your tablets! Occasionally two medicines are combined in a single tablet.

ACE inhibitors

ACE (angiotensin-converting enzyme) is a chemical produced naturally by the body. Its task is to make another chemical, called angiotensin, and this is responsible for constricting blood vessels and making the kidneys retain salt and water. Normally, more angiotensin is produced in response to some problem with the circulation – such as a large loss of blood or heart failure. The result is a vicious circle whereby blood vessels become more constricted, increasing the pressure on the heart, which causes the body to produce more angiotensin, and so on.

ACE inhibitors work by interrupting this cycle. In so doing, they relieve breathlessness and enable the person to be more active, but they also delay or prevent any further deterioration in heart function, helping people with heart failure to live longer. Sometimes they may need to be

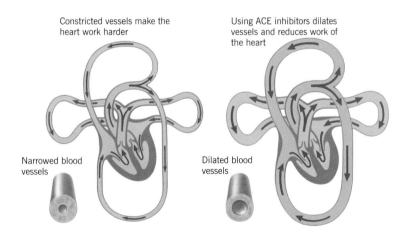

Constricted vessels make the heart work harder

Using ACE inhibitors dilates vessels and reduces work of the heart

Narrowed blood vessels

Dilated blood vessels

How ACE inhibitors affect your body.

taken in conjunction with water tablets if the person has fluid retention – swollen ankles, for example (see page 24).

As well as being used to treat heart failure, ACE inhibitors may also be prescribed for high blood pressure or to protect the heart following a heart attack.

As with any medicine, some people will experience side effects when taking ACE inhibitors, but these are mostly minor and usually wear off after a couple of weeks. Headaches and tiredness are the most common. More troublesome side effects can include dizziness and coughing; these can usually be overcome with a bit of help.

Dizziness is caused by a fall in blood pressure as the veins and arteries relax and this fall can occasionally trigger a blackout if the blood pressure isn't high enough to get blood up to the brain against gravity. It is most likely to happen to someone having their first dose if he or she has been taking large doses of diuretics (water tablets) for some time. This is why you may be advised to lie down after taking your first dose of ACE inhibitor. Anyone who is known to be at risk of a blackout may be asked to take their first dose under the supervision of a doctor or nurse, possibly in hospital.

Coughing is common in people with heart failure even when they aren't taking ACE inhibitors. A cough caused by the medicine is usually dry, ticklish and persistent, and may well stop you (or your partner) from sleeping. Some people find their cough is eased by taking sodium cromoglycate – a medicine often used in inhalers by children with asthma. For others, however, the cough is bad enough to prevent them from taking ACE inhibitors in which case angiotensin II blockers (see below) may be given.

Certain types of kidney disease may make it impossible for some people to take ACE inhibitors at all. Other patients with kidney problems may be alright provided they can come off other blood pressure-lowering medicines and water tablets, or can at least take ACE inhibitors in reduced doses. If you have kidney problems, your doctor will keep a close eye on you if you're taking ACE inhibitors.

Angiotensin II blockers
These agents block the effects of angiotensin II on the heart and blood vessels, effectively doing a similar job to ACE inhibitors. They do not cause cough. At the moment, these agents are generally reserved as an alternative to ACE inhibitors for patients who

MEDICAL TREATMENTS

Target of therapy	Medicine
Fluid retention	Diuretics
Relief of breathlessness	Diuretics/ACE inhibitors/beta-blockers
Heart protection	Beta-blockers/ACE inhibitors/spironolactone
Atrial fibrillation	Digoxin/beta-blockers/amiodarone
Blood clots	Warfarin

develop cough with ACE inhibitors. Recent evidence suggests that some patients may benefit from a combination of ACE inhibitors and angiotensin II blockers. Your doctor will be able to advise you whether this is a good idea for you.

Water tablets (or diuretics)

These are designed to force the kidneys to get rid of salt and water. As a result, they can help with symptoms such as breathlessness and swollen ankles which result from fluid waterlogging the tissues; however, they don't have any effect on other problems associated with heart failure as far as we know.

They are often prescribed for people whose heart failure is newly diagnosed because they work quickly and can do only good in the short term, whatever the actual cause of heart failure. Your GP can get you to start taking them to relieve breathlessness and swollen ankles while investigations are being organised to find out what is the root cause of your symptoms – in other words, why you have heart failure. Once you have a detailed diagnosis, ACE inhibitors can be prescribed if you need them.

The amount of urine you pass or the quantity of fluid that you retain can cause measurable changes in your weight. Each litre of urine weighs one kilogram (2.2 pounds). By weighing yourself every day at the same time, you can check the amount of water you're passing out of the body in your urine. If you find that you have gained more than 2–3 kilograms (4–6 pounds) in one week and you are also becoming short of breath, you should ask your doctor whether you need to increase your dose of water tablets. If you can't get to speak to him or her, take an extra tablet and talk to the doctor the following day.

On the other hand, an attack of diarrhoea that leaves you 2–3 kg lighter probably means you should cut out the water tablets for a few days until your weight is back to normal. Don't hesitate to ask your doctor's advice in situations like this – usually a brief telephone call will be enough to answer all your questions.

Anyone who is taking powerful water tablets for the first time should bear in mind that you may need to have easy access to a toilet for a few hours after your first dose. Usually, your urine production will be less dramatic after the first few doses, but it's a good idea to take them at least 4–6 hours before bedtime so you don't have to get up during the night. Should you have to be somewhere where you can't be sure of getting to a toilet easily, it is worth postponing taking the water tablet until a more convenient point in your day.

One important possible side effect of the more powerful diuretics is urinary retention in those men whose prostate gland is enlarged. The kidneys are stimulated by the tablets into producing urine much faster than usual causing the bladder to overfill. It is important to tell or remind your doctor if you have difficulty passing urine before you take any new water tablets.

Some people develop gout as a result of taking water tablets – the main symptom is usually a hot and painful big toe. This can be readily treated and subsequent attacks prevented by changing your tablets or adding an anti-gout medicine. (Gout is caused by uric acid in the following way: uric acid is normally present in the bloodstream and is filtered into the urine by the kidneys. Diuretics make the blood more concentrated, and some reduce the amount of uric acid in the urine. When the uric acid levels get high it crystallises out in the joints causing gout.)

You're likely to have regular blood tests at least every year to check for any sign that your kidneys are working less efficiently (if this happens you may need to have your tablets changed). If you're on ACE inhibitors as well as water tablets, dizziness is a possible side effect. If you do experience this, talk to your doctor who will probably reduce the dose of diuretics.

Most diuretics cause the body to lose a substance called potassium and this can lead to a feeling of weakness and rhythm upsets in the heart. Other diuretics can help the body hold on to potassium. Potassium-losing and -retaining diuretics are often given together to keep the potassium balance right. In some patients with severe heart failure, other types of diuretics may be used for additional effect – some of these can make you pass an awful lot of urine.

Spironolactone

This is a potassium-retaining diuretic that blocks the effects of a hormone called aldosterone. Aldosterone is increased in patients with heart failure and, although treatment with ACE inhibitors reduces aldosterone levels, they are not completely effective in this respect. In patients taking large doses of conventional tablets (for example, two or more tablets of frusemide per day), the addition of spironolactone has been shown to delay deterioration of the heart and help patients with heart failure to live longer.

Beta-blockers

In combination with ACE inhibitors, beta-blockers are the most effective treatment for most patients with heart failure.

Beta-blockers block the effects of the chemical messenger adrenaline on the heart, blood vessels and also the lungs. Adrenaline causes the heart to beat faster, and also to pump more strongly. In the lungs, adrenaline causes the main airways to relax and widen. This is why beta-blockers can be dangerous in people with asthma. Beta-blockers lower the blood pressure and in the short term the pumping strength of the heart. They are widely prescribed to control high blood pressure and are often very effective. However, because they reduce the pumping strength of the heart, doctors have avoided giving these medicines to people with heart failure for many years. Newer evidence suggests that, started in very small doses and increased slowly, they may be remarkably effective in reducing symptoms, strengthening the heart (in the long term) and helping people with heart failure to live longer. At the moment, experts disagree about whether this applies to all beta-blockers or just to certain ones, such as carvedilol, bisoprolol and metoprolol.

Side effects are not uncommon when starting a beta-blocker. Dizziness, fatigue and increased breathlessness may be encountered. Diabetic patients may notice that their blood sugar tends to run higher. With time side effects usually resolve and after 2–3 months the benefits of beta-blockade begin to appear. Some patients can respond dramatically but it takes time! In a few cases, beta-blockers may even cure heart failure. However, patience is required.

The doses of beta-blocker should be increased gradually at

two- to four-weekly intervals over a period of months to achieve maintenance doses. Increasing the dose more quickly often leads to problems.

Beta-blockers may also be used to control atrial fibrillation.

Digoxin

This is the purified form of digitalis, which was made for centuries from foxgloves. Treatment in tablet form is rather more reliable than the old herbal preparations, which poisoned as many people as they helped. Although digoxin in its natural form was discovered by an Englishman called William Withering over 200 years ago, we still don't know how it works nor are we sure how useful it really is. Popular tradition suggests that it strengthens weakened heart muscle, but we don't know whether this actually is the way it helps. At least it does appear to relieve symptoms. It is certainly effective at controlling the heart rate, which is why it is the most popular choice for treating those people whose heart failure is caused by atrial fibrillation. Doctors disagree about whether digoxin should be prescribed for people whose heart rhythm is regular – some think it should be reserved only for particularly difficult cases.

Of all the tablets prescribed for heart failure, digoxin is probably the one with the fewest side effects when taken in the appropriate dose, but if it builds up in the body it can be dangerous. The body gets rid of it very slowly, which is why it is taken only once a day. Once you stop taking it, it is about a week before all traces of it disappear from your system. Older people (aged 75 or over) and anyone with kidney problems can only take digoxin in small doses. Too much of it may provoke feelings of nausea and vomiting, and some people start seeing everything tinged with yellow; older people may become confused. Anyone who suspects that they have developed any of these side effects should stop taking digoxin and contact their doctor for advice.

Nitrates

These medicines are frequently taken by people with angina, but they may also be useful for people with heart failure who can't take ACE inhibitors. Nitrates work by relaxing the blood vessels. This makes it easier for the heart to pump blood out into the circulation and also lowers the pressure of the blood draining back to the heart. Nitrates also open up the blood vessels which take oxygen to the heart muscle itself, which helps it to work as well as possible.

HOW ARE MEDICINES GIVEN?

- **Swallowed:** as tablets or capsules
- **Sublingual:** tablet is placed under the tongue until it dissolves
- **Buccal:** held between the upper gum and lip
- **Aerosol spray:** directly into the mouth
- **Self-adhesive patch:** the medicine in the patch is absorbed through skin directly into the bloodstream
- **Intravenously:** rapidly injected directly into a vein or more slowly through an intravenous drip
- **Intramuscularly:** injection deep into a muscle mass, e.g. the buttock
- **Subcutaneously:** underneath the skin

However, there is little evidence that nitrates make an important difference to symptoms or the underlying heart problem. The patient or doctor may wish to try and see if it makes a difference on a case-to-case basis.

Nitrates, for angina, can be taken in several different ways: as a spray used under the tongue, or as tablets to be dissolved between the gums and cheek.

Nitrates are also available as skin patches. The medicine is in the patch, which looks like transparent plaster, and is absorbed through the skin into the circulation. The medicine does not work directly on the heart so there is no advantage in putting the patch on the skin over your heart, but some people like the idea!

Aspirin

Aspirin makes the blood less likely to clot. Platelets in the blood start off clot formation which can end up as a heart attack or stroke. Aspirin makes the platelets less sticky. However, there is doubt as to whether it actually produces much benefit for people whose major problem is heart failure.

Aspirin can irritate the lining of the stomach making it more likely to bleed. It also interferes with warfarin in the circulation and can result in the blood becoming too thin. You should double-check with your doctor before taking aspirin and warfarin together.

Warfarin

This stops blood clots forming in areas of the heart where the circulation is sluggish (if, for example, you have atrial fibrillation, see page 16). If clots form, bits may break off and be pumped out into the circulation where they can become lodged in smaller vessels. If a clot gets stuck in an artery supplying an area of the brain it will cause a stroke. If it ends up in an artery to, for example, the leg, then it will cause severe pain and, untreated, gangrene may develop.

While you're taking warfarin, you will need regular blood tests to make sure that you are on the correct dose. Warfarin interacts with many other medicines, so you should always remind any doctor you see that you are taking it. You also have to be careful about over-the-counter medicines, especially aspirin – ask for advice from your doctor or the pharmacist before taking anything new. If you enjoy alcohol, keep your consumption to sensible levels and avoid binge drinking. Warfarin is broken down in the liver. Alcohol increases the rate at which warfarin is broken down by the liver, by speeding up the liver enzymes. If the amount of alcohol you drink varies widely then so will the clotting ability of your blood.

Amiodarone
This medicine is a very effective

way of controlling abnormal heart rhythms and can restore a regular rhythm to those with atrial fibrillation, sometimes when other treatments haven't worked. Unfortunately, some people can't take it because of side effects. The most common is sensitisation to sunlight, which is a particular problem for people with fair skins. It can take up to a year for the problem to become apparent, so it's important to take care when in the sun and ask your doctor for advice immediately if you are at all concerned. It is also possible for it to cause the thyroid gland to become overactive, so if you start losing weight rapidly, a sign of thyroid overactivity, while on amiodarone, see your doctor who will arrange a blood test.

More serious side effects can occur in the liver and lungs because amiodarone can cause jaundice and shortness of breath, but these side effects are rare in people taking less than 400 milligrams a day.

For those people who don't experience these side effects, however, amiodarone can be a very effective treatment.

Calcium channel blockers
People who have angina or high blood pressure may be treated with calcium channel blockers. These

Class of drug	Generic/scientific name	Comments
ACE inhibitors	Captopril	
	Cilazapril	
	Enalapril	
	Fosinopril	
	Lisinopril	
	Perindopril	
	Quinapril	
	Ramipril	
	Trandolapril	
Angiotensin II blockers	Candesartan	
	Irbesartan	
	Losartan	
	Valsartan	
Diuretics	Amiloride	For patients with severe heart failure even powerful diuretics may lose their effectiveness. This can often be restored by combining a thiazide and a powerful diuretic
	Bendrofluazide	
	Bumetanide	
	Chlorothiazide	
	Chlorthalidone	
	Frusemide	
	Hydrochlorothiazide	
	Metolazone	
	Spironolactone	Spironolactone may be especially effective in preventing worsening of heart failure when used in conjunction with other ACE inhibitors
	Torasemide	
	Triamterene	
	Xipamide	
Beta-blockers	Bisoprolol	Bisoprolol, carvedilol and metoprolol are beta-blockers that are proven to be effective in heart failure
	Carvedilol	
	Labetalol	
	Metoprolol	Carvedilol is approved for the treatment of heart failure
	Propranolol	
	Sotalol	
	Timolol	
Cardiac glycosides	Digoxin	
Nitrates + nitrate-like medicines	Glyceryl trinitrate	These medications should be used with care in patients with heart failure. Whether they are needed or not should be kept under continuous review
	Isosorbide dinitrate	
	Isosorbide mononitrate	
	Nicorandil	
	Pentaerythritol tetranitrate	
Calcium channel blockers	Amlodipine	
	Diltiazem	
	Felodipine	
	Isradipine	
	Lacidipine	
	Nicardipine	
	Nifedipine	
	Nisoldipine	
	Verapamil	
Alpha-blockers	Doxazosin	These medications should be used with care in patients with heart failure. Whether they are needed or not should be kept under continuous re
	Indoramin	
	Prazosin	
	Terazosin	
Antiplatelets	Abciximab	
	Aspirin	
	Clopidogrel	
	Dipyridamole	
Anticoagulants	Heparin	Correct dosage is very important
	Warfarin	

Pharmaceutical companies all give their products 'proprietary/trade' names as well as their actual 'generic/scien.
You will be able to find this on the package of your medication.

ype	Purpose	Possible side effects for class of drug
	To improve symptoms and to try to prevent worsening heart failure	Persistent dry cough, dizziness
	To try to prevent worsening heart failure (less evidence than for ACE inhibitors)	Headache, dizziness (not associated with cough)
ₒtassium sparing ıiazide diuretic ₒwerful diuretic ıiazide diuretic ₒtassium sparing ₒwerful diuretic ıiazide diuretic ıiazide diuretic ₒtassium sparing ₒwerful diuretic ₒtassium sparing ıiazide diuretic	Force the kidneys to get rid of salt and water	Gout, dramatic increase in urine production Can lead to urine retention in men with an enlarged prostate
		Tiredness, lethargy, cold hands, nightmares
	Regulates heart rate	Excess can lead to nausea, vomiting and confusion
	Relieve angina	Faintness, throbbing headache, dizziness and flushing
	Relieve angina, reduce blood pressure (BP)	Flushing, headache, ankle swelling, constipation
	Relieve angina, reduce BP	Headache, dizziness, vomiting
	Reduce BP	Fainting, fluid retention
	Thin blood	Gastric upset
	Prevent blood clots forming in the circulation	Care must be taken with possible interactions with other medicines

e. Only the generic name is listed here.

medicines block the action of calcium on the heart muscle and blood vessels. Calcium channel blockers reduce the amount of calcium entering the muscle cells of the coronary arteries and other blood vessels in the circulation, causing them to relax and open up. This increases the blood supply to the heart and reduces the work the heart has to do to pump blood round the circulatory system. These are good effects in treating angina and high blood pressure.

However, a possible side effect is that the heart may pump less powerfully, making the heart failure worse and causing the body to retain more salt and water. Newer calcium channel blockers, such as amlodipine, seem to be safe and may be used in patients with heart failure to treat angina or high blood pressure.

CARDIOVERSION

Cardioversion is the medical term for correcting an abnormal heart rhythm using an electric shock. This is always done in hospital, either under a general anaesthetic or, less often, under heavy sedation. The electric shock disrupts the heart's abnormal electrical rhythm allowing a normal rhythm to take over again in many cases.

The procedure only takes minutes and the benefits in terms of improved heart function are clear

soon afterwards. Some people have to keep taking medical treatment to reduce the chances of the abnormal rhythm recurring. Warfarin may also be prescribed before cardioversion to prevent clots from the heart being released into the circulation once the heart is pumping normally again (see page 40).

SURGICAL TREATMENT

If the problem with the heart is structural – a leaky valve or blocked blood vessel, for example – surgery may be possible. For a more complete explanation of surgical treatments see the Family Doctor book *Understanding Heart Surgery*.

Faulty valves

If the valve is too narrow, it is sometimes possible to stretch it, but if it's leaking it will have to be repaired or replaced. Replacement valves are of two main types: either synthetic, made of metal and plastic, or biological, taken from pigs. These days valve surgery is commonplace and, although it is still a major operation, the success rates are good.

Narrowed blood vessels

Narrowed blood vessels to the heart muscle may cause angina and heart attacks. It used to be thought that a heart attack always destroyed heart muscle leaving behind a scar.

Recently, it has become clear that heart attacks may just stun heart muscle or put it into a long-term sleep (often termed hibernation). Medical treatment, especially beta-blockers, or a procedure to improve the blood supply to the heart may revive sleeping heart muscle. Experts disagree whether pills or one of the procedures below is the safest and most effective way to treat this problem. The British government is running a large study to help doctors decide how future patients are best treated.

• **Coronary artery bypass graft (CABG):** When coronary arteries (which are the vessels supplying blood to the heart muscle) are blocked or narrowed, too little blood may reach the heart muscle, which stops it contracting properly. In this situation, a coronary bypass operation may be needed. This restores a normal blood supply usually by using a vein from the leg to bypass the blocked sections of coronary artery. Coronary bypass grafting is a major operation, but thousands of people benefit from it every year. Most only have to stay in hospital for a week or 10 days.

• **Angioplasty:** Sometimes, a narrowed artery can be opened by a procedure called angioplasty. This involves passing a narrow tube (called a catheter) into the obstructed artery. Around the catheter is a small balloon which is expanded in the narrowed area. It clears the obstruction, opening up

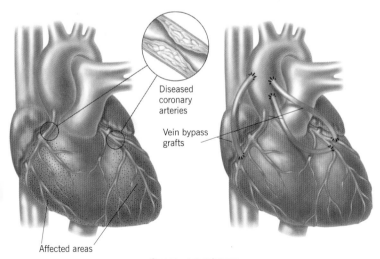

Diseased coronary arteries

Vein bypass grafts

Affected areas

Coronary artery bypass.

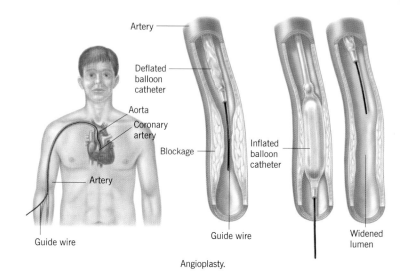

Artery

Deflated balloon catheter

Aorta

Coronary artery

Blockage

Inflated balloon catheter

Artery

Guide wire

Guide wire

Widened lumen

Angioplasty.

the artery so blood can flow through it properly. Experts are working on the development of other devices designed to achieve an even better result than a balloon. However, angioplasty is not suitable for everyone with narrowed blood vessels (angioplasty is less successful if there are multiple blockages), and thorough investigations including catheter tests and heart scans (see page 30) are necessary before the decision is made to use it.

Aneurysmectomy

This procedure involves removing the healed scar after a severe heart attack in the hope that this will improve the heart's efficiency. In carefully selected patients this can be quite successful.

Pacemakers

The muscle of the heart is stimulated to contract by a complex 'wiring' system. When the heart is badly damaged the electrical conduction system within the heart, which controls and triggers heart muscle contraction, may also be damaged, leading to heart 'block' and this may lead to the heart going too slowly. The patient may notice a worsening of heart failure or blackouts if this happens. A pacemaker can do much the same job as the heart's own wiring system, although never quite as well. A pacemaker consists of a battery about the size of a matchbox (the battery life is usually many years), which can be inserted under the skin with a small operation, usually under a local anaesthetic.

Wires can then be attached to the battery and threaded through the veins to stimulate the heart.

More recently it has been realised that damage to the heart's own wiring system may lead some parts of the surviving heart muscle to contract while other parts are relaxing. This lack of synchrony leads to a further loss of the efficiency of the heart. A device such as a pacemaker can be used to stimulate the heart in a synchronous (coordinated) fashion, increasing its efficiency. This is a promising new treatment that is available only in a few specialist centres. It is not yet clear precisely how useful this treatment is, but the results of large studies should be available by 2003.

Implantable defibrillators

Some patients may have serious upsets of their heart rhythm which could cause blackouts or may indicate that there is a high risk of a cardiac arrest. A defibrillator is similar to a pacemaker (but a little larger), which can give the heart an electric shock if a serious rhythm upset occurs (similar to a cardioversion for atrial fibrillation – see page 44). These devices are available only in specialist centres. Patients require intensive investigation by a specialist to ascertain whether they are suitable for such treatment.

Transplantation

This may be an option for younger people with severe heart failure. It is often less useful for people over the age of 60 or so, because they may well have widespread artery disease that makes surgery complicated and means they do less well in the long term. The operation does involve risk, but around 85 per cent of people survive the first month after surgery, and 75 per cent will still be alive five years later.

After surgery, patients who undergo transplantation have to take powerful medicines to prevent their immune systems from rejecting their new heart. As a result of this immune suppression, they are prone to serious infections. They also need regular tests and biopsies (a technique for picking off a small piece of heart muscle) to check that their new hearts are working properly. Although heart transplantation can be very successful for the right person, it is not a cure.

For many people with mild heart failure, medical treatment is better than a transplant. In any case, the number of transplants possible is severely limited by the number of donor hearts available. Around 400 operations are done in this country each year; more than 100,000 people develop heart failure over the same period.

KEY POINTS

✓ Most patients require treatment with ACE inhibitors, beta-blockers and diuretics

✓ If atrial fibrillation is present, most patients also require digoxin and warfarin

How to help yourself

Although you may depend on your regular medicines to keep you feeling well and active, there is plenty you can do to help yourself and maximise the benefit you get from your treatment. Some of the lifestyle changes suggested here may seem difficult, especially at first, but the rewards will come in a greater sense of well-being and important health benefits.

WAYS TO BOOST YOUR WELL-BEING

Smoking

Anyone who smokes already knows that it is bad for their health, but people with heart failure are taking serious extra risks by continuing to smoke:

- It makes it more likely that you will have (another) heart attack, so damaging the heart muscle more and making heart failure worse. If you give up smoking after having a heart attack, you halve your chances of having another one.

- Smoking contributes to the development of coronary artery disease. It seems to promote the build-up of cholesterol, make the blood stickier and lower levels of substances in the blood that help protect your arteries from clogging.

- Smokers have lower levels of oxygen in their blood than non-smokers and, as we've seen, diminished oxygen supply to the heart and body is already a problem for people with heart failure anyway.

- Smoking causes progressive damage to the lungs.

The more you smoke the worse it is but one cigarette constricts the blood vessels, including those in the heart, for 18 hours! The best solution is to give up smoking completely.

Diet

You may need to think in terms of a weight-reducing diet if you're overweight because weight puts an extra strain on your heart. Otherwise, it's more a question of

SALT SENSE

Your doctor will probably advise you in particular to be wary about the amount of salt you consume. Unless you are told specifically to do so, you don't need to try to follow a salt-free diet, which can be pretty tasteless. It's usually enough just to cut down on any foods that are very high in salt – which includes some that you wouldn't immediately suspect, so get into the habit of checking food labels. Ordinary salt may be listed as sodium chloride. Generally salt substitutes are not recommended as they are usually potassium chloride which may interact with some heart failure medications such as water tablets and ACE inhibitors.

High salt foods

- Most canned foods (except fruit)
- Most canned and packet soups
- Sausages (including hot dogs, salami, etc.)
- Pickled foods

- Salted nuts, crisps and cheesy biscuits
- Pizza and many other fast foods
- Many Chinese and other Oriental dishes

Low salt foods

- Most breakfast cereals, bread and pasta
- Fresh white or oily fish (not smoked fish or shellfish)
- Fruit and vegetables (check can labels for salt)

- Herbs, spices, lemon juice and other non-salt seasonings
- Semi-skimmed milk, plain yoghurt
- Fresh meat and poultry

adjusting your diet to make sure it's as healthy as possible. This is likely to mean cutting down on the fat content, especially saturated fats which mostly come from animal sources, for example, cheese, butter, eggs, biscuits and cakes. You should also aim to have several servings of fresh vegetables, fruit and salad every day and plenty of natural fibre from other sources such as wholemeal bread and cereals, rice and pasta.

Traditionally, the British diet has not included a wide range of pulses – apart from baked beans – but they are a good source of protein and fibre. If you already enjoy Asian cooking, you will know all about the many delicious pulse-based dishes such as dhal, although you should be wary of high salt content in restaurant or prepared dishes (see Salt sense, on page 50).

When cooking at home, it's worth putting peas and the many different kinds of beans as well as lentils on the menu more often. If you feel you could use some specific advice on how to improve your diet, ask to see a dietitian either at the health centre or at the hospital.

Before you conclude that you do need to lose weight, you need to allow for any fluid retention that might be making you seem overweight when you really are not. Rather than try to work it out for yourself, it's probably best to talk it over with your doctor, who will help you to decide whether you should lose weight. If so, you can also get advice on your target weight and the most sensible way to set about reaching it.

Alcohol

You may have been told that too much alcohol has caused damage to your heart muscle; in that case, total abstinence is the only sensible course. Otherwise, alcohol in moderation should do no harm, provided you avoid 'binge' drinking.

Rest and exercise

Although you may need to rest in bed if your heart failure is severe or while your treatment is being stabilised, exercise is generally good for you.

Whenever you can, make a point of getting some kind of exercise each day. A brisk walk uphill or round the park is probably the best choice. When the weather is too bad or it's difficult to get out for some reason, then making the beds or doing other housework at a smart pace is sufficiently demanding. There are, however, some forms of exercise that you shouldn't try.

TAKING YOUR MEDICATION

Tablets only work if you take them. They do you no good in the bottle. However well intentioned you may be, it can be difficult to remember to take them, so if you have a problem, work out some way of reminding yourself or checking whether you have taken them. For example, you could set your watch alarm for the appropriate time, or get hold of a proper pill dispenser from the pharmacy. Alternatively, make a simple one for yourself from an egg box – just set out your day's dose each morning then you can check later whether you've taken them.

Remember that you may need to retime your water tablets if you're going to be out and away from a toilet for some time. You should also plan to take them several hours before you go to bed. Other tablets should be taken at around the same time each day so as to keep the level of the medicine in your blood as constant as possible.

Should you notice any side effects from any of the medicines you are taking, discuss the matter with your doctor. There are alternatives available in most cases, and sometimes it needs a bit of trial and error to find which ones suit you best. Make sure you organise a new supply before the old one runs out and that you always have enough to cover you for holidays.

CHECKING YOUR PROGRESS

When you start treatment, you should notice an improvement in your symptoms. Breathlessness in particular should become less of a problem. You should also find you can gradually do a bit more as far as exercise is concerned as your stamina starts to come back. Water tablets usually improve symptoms quickly. ACE inhibitors may take weeks and beta-blockers months to have their full effects. You may feel temporarily worse for a week or so after starting a beta-blocker.

How you get on doing the same task is a useful gauge of how well your heart is working. Aim to set yourself at least one task to do three or four times a week – something that gets you mildly out of breath, like walking uphill to the shops. Don't overdo it so that you end up completely puffed. If at any time you notice yourself getting more out of breath doing the same walk or that you seem to be able to do less and less, report this to your doctor.

Don't forget, however, that other illnesses could also be playing a part: for example, a chest infection will make you breathless and you'll feel tired after you've had the flu.

Watch your weight

When heart failure is going out of control, relatively rapid weight change can occur and it's important that it's picked up as soon as possible. The point of weighing yourself each day is to check whether you are retaining too much fluid. You may recall from an earlier chapter (see page 36) that one litre of urine weighs one kilogram (that is, 2.2 lb) so any sudden weight gain indicates that you may be retaining fluid. Tell your doctor if you gain more than 2–3 kg (5–6 lb) in a week. It sounds obvious, but you do need to be sure you have a good, reliable set of bathroom scales and that they are standing on an even surface. You can't monitor your

weight accurately otherwise. Remember too that, if you're away from home and using different scales, the readings will almost certainly vary from the ones at home. The solution is to weigh yourself when you arrive at your destination if possible so you have a reference point against which to check any ups and downs in your weight. The best time for your daily weigh-in is first thing, before getting dressed but after emptying your bladder. You should note your weight each day in a diary. Normally, you'll find that your weight varies very little from one day to the next, even if the long-term trend is up or down.

What makes heart failure worse?

There are a number of reasons why someone with heart failure may find that their condition is gradually getting worse:

- Forgetting to take medication.
- Too much salt in the diet.
- Taking one or more medicines that can aggravate the problem, such as some treatments for arthritis and some painkillers. This includes some that you can buy without a prescription, such as ibuprofen, so always check with the pharmacist before buying anything you haven't used before.

He or she will usually be able to suggest acceptable alternatives – paracetamol rather than ibuprofen, for example. Some prescription medicines which you may have been taking for another heart condition – such as calcium channel blockers – may not be appropriate when you develop heart failure as they can make it worse. Do check with your doctor if you are still taking them.

- The condition which originally caused your heart failure starts to get worse.
- You develop some new problem with your heart, for example, if your heart rhythm becomes irregular, you may suddenly start feeling much worse and need new treatment.
- Infections, usually in the chest or urine.

WARNING SIGNS – AND WHAT TO DO

Chest pain

If you develop a crushing pain in your chest or down your arms and up into your jaw, rest in a sitting position. If you have GTN tablets to put under your tongue or a spray, ask someone to bring them to you if possible and use them immediately. If the pain hasn't gone after ten minutes, call an ambulance.

Palpitations

If you develop a fluttering feeling in your chest or feel your heart beating irregularly, rest for a while. If the feeling persists or happens often, you should see your doctor. You may have occasional extra beats known as ectopics or intermittent atrial fibrillation (see page 16) and may need treatment.

Breathlessness

- **Sudden**: If you wake up in the night severely short of breath, sit up and try to relax as much as you can. If symptoms do not settle quickly, contact your doctor or, if he or she can't be reached within five minutes, phone the ambulance. You have probably got extra fluid on the lungs which needs to be treated promptly with an increased dose of diuretic medication, probably in the form of an injection.

You may also need to be given oxygen.

- **Gradual**: If you find your physical activity becoming increasingly limited and your breathlessness increasing, see your doctor. You may need to have your medication adjusted or to try a different treatment.

Weight gain

This may be a sign of increased fluid retention if it happens over a relatively short time, for example, 2–3 kg (5–6 lb) in a week or so (see page 53). See your doctor as you'll probably need to increase your dose of water tablets.

Dizziness

This can be a side effect of some medications, especially ACE inhibitors. You may be able to prevent it if you always remember to get up from lying down or sitting in stages – for example, when you're getting up in the morning, sit on the side of the bed for a few minutes before you stand up. This prevents your blood pressure from dropping suddenly. Should you have a dizzy spell or feel faint, lie down.

It may help if you raise your legs a little by resting them on cushions or on a chair. See your doctor if dizziness persists or if you have a blackout. Adjusting your medication may improve matters.

Discuss this with your doctor or nurse first. For most patients who are not severely breathless a reduction in the dose of water tablets is worth a try. If weight increases by more than two to three pounds (one to one and a half kilograms) or breathlessness or ankle swelling get worse, then you should restart treatment immediately and see your doctor.

KEY POINTS

✓ Don't smoke

✓ Eat a healthy diet (avoid excess salt)

✓ Take a sensible amount of exercise

✓ Take your medicines accurately

✓ Weigh yourself (and note) regularly

Living with heart failure

Anyone who has a condition like heart failure which usually cannot be completely cured will gradually learn from experience how they can best cope with it. As a general rule, the more you understand about what is wrong and why you get the symptoms you do, the more you can help to minimise them, even if they can't be prevented altogether.

You need to know what has caused your heart failure, or how it's being treated, and the purpose of any medication you are taking. Do you know the right time of day to take it and what side effects, if any, to watch for? Make sure you are clear about when and in what circumstances you need to call your doctor, other than for routine appointments.

It helps enormously if you can build up a good relationship with your GP and with any specialist who's treating you. It is important for you to feel you can ask any questions you want and contact the doctors for advice when you feel in need of it. You can help them to help you by not missing appointments unnecessarily, and possibly keeping notes of any questions, minor changes in your condition or your response to treatment so you don't forget anything when you next see them.

Your doctors have to rely on you to let them know how you are doing on a day-to-day basis – which is why it's important to get into the habit of monitoring your condition. This means regular daily weigh-ins as outlined on page 53, as well as noting any changes in how much you can do or in other symptoms.

You will feel the benefit of regular daily exercise – enough to leave you feeling mildly breathless, but not too much so. Doing something like a brisk walk every day is ideal, but try to manage some exercise at least three times a week if you can.

Depending on how you lived before you developed heart failure, you may need to give some thought to the amount of stress in your life and how you deal with it. Few of us can avoid stressful situations entirely, but it may be possible to reduce your exposure to it to some extent. Even if you can't do that much to get rid of the sources of stress, you can learn to handle it without getting too het up and tense. Many local education authorities run day-time or evening classes in relaxation or stress management and you can also buy cassettes designed to promote relaxation.

It cannot be said too often that smoking can only add to your problems if you have heart failure, so the effort involved in giving up is well worth while. Do ask your doctor for practical advice as well as the addresses and telephone numbers of organisations which can give you information and support when you want to stop smoking. Your doctor should also be able to fill any gaps in your knowledge about the right kind of diet or arrange for you to have a chat with a dietitian if necessary. Eating properly can give a boost to your overall health, even if you don't need to worry about losing weight. And if you could do with shedding some excess fat, it's sensible to get a dietitian's advice on how to lose it slowly without going hungry or missing out on essential nutrients. Remember that carrying too much extra weight puts added strain on your heart, and makes any kind of exercise even more difficult than it might otherwise be.

Having heart failure doesn't mean you have to give up all your former pleasures, however! Unless your heart failure was actually the result of damage caused by excessive drinking, you don't have to give up alcohol. Moderate drinking won't do any harm, although beer drinkers may need to watch the volume of liquid they consume if they are prone to fluid retention.

Some people are also concerned that their heart problem may curtail their sex life. In fact, the only aspect of heart failure that might affect your ability to make love is being short of breath. Otherwise, there is no reason why you shouldn't have sex whenever you and your partner feel like it. The only exception is during the period immediately after a heart attack, when you should abstain from sex for about six weeks to allow the heart to heal.

SELF-MONITORING

Get into the habit of monitoring your condition. Weigh yourself and note any changes in how you feel or how much you can do on a daily basis. Photocopy or make and complete a weekly chart like this:

Week no. [　　　]

Date	Weight (Early morning, empty bladder)	How I feel (At the end of the day)

Medicine name	Dose	Frequency

SELF-MONITORING

Get into the habit of monitoring your condition. Weigh yourself and note any changes in how you feel or how much you can do on a daily basis. Photocopy or make and complete a weekly chart like this:

Week no. [ ]

Date	Weight (Early morning, empty bladder)	How I feel (At the end of the day)

Medicine name	Dose	Frequency

TRAVEL AND HOLIDAYS

If you're planning a long journey or stay away from home, it's a good idea to have a word with your doctor beforehand. Anyone travelling outside the UK needs good travel insurance. You may find that many of the standard policies don't cover you for conditions that you already know about when you take them out – such as heart failure. Should you encounter difficulties, contact the British Heart Foundation (address on page 71) who can give you a list of insurance companies sympathetic to those with heart complaints. Before you leave home, you should also check with your GP whether you need any immunisations or to take tablets to help protect you against malaria, for example.

Unless your heart failure is severe, your doctor will probably encourage you in your plans and suggest any precautions you need to take to maintain optimum fitness. You will need to take particular care if your destination is very hot or very cold, and people with more than mild heart failure are normally advised not to visit high-altitude resorts – those over 2,000 metres (6,000 feet) – because there is less oxygen in the atmosphere. You needn't be put off by the prospect of long flights or journeys by other means and even extremes of temperature, however, provided you plan ahead and follow some commonsense rules while you're away.

How to travel

Having decided on your destination, you may or may not have any real choice about what means of transport you use to get there. When you do have options, however, or the journey is a factor in choosing where to go, you need to work out your priorities. For example, a car is the ideal choice if your main concern is to be able to travel at your own pace and stop whenever you want. On the other hand, long journeys by car can be stressful, especially if you're the only driver. Trains and even coaches have toilets on board and you can get up and stretch your legs if you want. Travelling by sea is relaxing – provided you're not prone to seasickness! If you are, it's worth taking antihistamine patches with you or wearing them all the time you're on board if necessary. Remember that sickness can lead to a reduction in your salt and fluid levels and prevent you absorbing medication, so it's important to avoid it if you can.

Flying may be the most convenient as well as the fastest way to your destination, but airports can be very stressful as well as involving long treks to the departure gates. The level of oxygen in aircraft cabins is lower than normal, but this is not usually a problem unless heart failure is severe. On long flights, you must take care not to become dehydrated, especially if you are taking diuretic tablets or ACE inhibitors. You should steer clear of alcohol as it increases the risk of dehydration and try to move around the aircraft at least once every hour or so if you can to stop blood clots forming in the legs. It's a wise precaution to let the airline know that you have heart failure, if it is severe, when you book so that they can make supplementary oxygen available just in case. You can also book a wheelchair if you need it, and

HOLIDAY CHECKPOINTS

- Talk to your doctor before you go and discuss how to tackle potential problems. In particular, make sure you understand what to do if your weight increases or drops suddenly while you're away.

- Make sure you have adequate health insurance cover and that it does not exclude 'pre-existing' conditions such as heart failure.

- Check that scales will be available at your destination and, if not, consider making room for a set in your luggage.

- If you're travelling by sea or air, let the airline or shipping company know that you have heart failure when you book.

- Keep a close eye on your weight while you're away and be prepared to adjust your medication, salt and fluid intake in case of any sudden changes.

- Take sensible precautions to protect your health – don't overdo the alcohol and steer clear of any food or drink liable to provoke tummy upsets. In countries where hygiene standards may be dubious, avoid ice cream, shellfish, fruit that needs washing rather than peeling, and salads and ice (unless from bottled water).

- Always protect your skin against the sun and, if taking amiodarone, apply a total block before going out in the sun.

most UK airports now offer a buggy service to get you to the plane if necessary, but you need to check whether this is also available at your destination airport.

When you arrive

As soon as you can after you arrive, you need to weigh yourself. Either check in advance with the hotel or pack your own scales (provided that there is someone else to carry your bag!). You may well find the result is different from your home scales, so use this as your reference point – all scales vary. You may be eating quite a different diet from usual, so you need to keep an eye on your salt and fluid balance. Continue to weigh yourself daily, and if your weight drops by more than 3 kg, you'll need to take action. It means that you are short of fluid, so if you're on water tablets, stop taking them for the time being. Otherwise, eat salty foods – such as nuts and crisps – and drink lots of non-alcoholic fluids until your weight is within 2–3 kg of your target weight.

Remember that if you have a tummy upset with diarrhoea and/or vomiting, you can easily become dehydrated. If severe, you need to stop taking water tablets and ACE inhibitors for a while, and drink lots of non-alcoholic drinks. Keep weighing yourself until the scales tell you your fluid balance is nearly back to normal, when you can restart your usual medicines. Don't hesitate to see a local doctor if you don't feel able to handle the situation on your own. Remember that vomiting, diarrhoea and sweating can also lead to salt depletion, which may lead to muscle cramps.

Sunburn – and even a suntan – is a sign that your skin is being damaged by exposure to the sun. All of us need to cover up and use sun protection products whenever we're out in good weather, but this is even more important for anyone taking amiodarone. The longer you've been taking it, the more likely it is that it will accumulate in your skin causing light sensitivity. Ordinary suntan products won't be sufficient to protect you against amiodarone sunburn, and you'll need to use a total sunblock as well as wearing a sunhat and cover-up clothes.

YOUR FAMILY AND FRIENDS

Family and friends can't help being concerned about your condition, but they may worry less if they can learn more about it. Obviously, individuals vary as to how much detail they want to know. The last thing you need from those close to you is gloom and doom, and they will find it far easier to adopt a positive approach when they know something about your condition and treatment. You will probably rely on their moral support on days when you are feeling less well so the more they understand the better. Most people want the answers to a few basic questions.

What is heart failure?

The term sounds rather dramatic and some people think it means your heart is going to stop any moment now. It will probably help to read the introductory section on pages 1–4.

How does it affect you?

People you spend a lot of time with or see regularly need to know about any limitations that your condition places on you. For example, the fact that you can't perhaps walk as far or as fast as you once did or can no longer do heavy gardening or carry heavy shopping.

Will it get worse?

Most people with heart failure find it easier to cope if they have someone they can rely on if they get new symptoms or old ones return, explain what symptoms could affect you, such as increased breathlessness or problems with your fluid balance, and what needs doing in a given set of circumstances. It can also be a big help if someone else remembers to check that you have taken your medicines as and when you should!

What should a relative or friend do in an emergency?

It may never happen, but someone who has been on a first aid course that includes basic resuscitation techniques will feel much more confident about coping in a crisis. A basic 'save-a-life' course takes only two hours. If they know what to do when someone loses consciousness while waiting for the ambulance, they could save someone's life one day! Contact the St John Ambulance (see page 72) or the Red Cross.

Who is at risk?

Knowing that you have heart failure may lead your relatives to worry whether they may develop the same problem one day. Anyone who is worried should explain the situation to their doctor, giving as much information about your condition as possible. The GP will then be able to advise them as to whether they need any investigations.

It may be necessary for close family members to have regular blood pressure or cholesterol checks, and they may be told that smoking presents even greater risks for them than for others. In some cases, relatives will need to have ECGs or echocardiography (see pages 28 and 29). However, it's quite likely that they will be

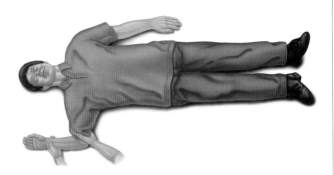

1. (a) Kneel beside the casualty.

   (b) Remove spectacles and any bulky items from pockets.

   (c) Straighten legs.

   (d) Place the arm nearest to you at right angles to the body.

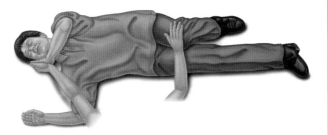

2. (a) Bring the arm furthest from you across the casualty's chest and hold the back of his hand against the cheek nearest to you.

   (b) Using your other hand, grasp the furthest leg just above the knee and raise it up until the foot is flat on the floor.

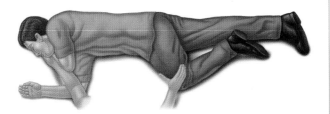

3. Keeping the casualty's hand pressed against his cheek, pull on the far leg and roll him towards you and on to his side.

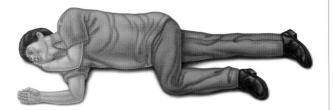

4. (a) Adjust the upper leg so that both the knee and hip are bent at right angles.

   (b) Tilt the head back to ensure the airway remains open.

   (c) Ensure the hand remains under the cheek, helping to keep the airway open.

told that their risk of developing heart failure is not increased just because you have it.

LOOKING TO THE FUTURE

The outlook for someone with heart failure will vary depending on what has caused it. For example, when it is the result of atrial fibrillation or valve disease, the underlying problem can often be cured so that the individual's prospects are similar to those of anyone else of around the same age. When the cause cannot be corrected in this way, the outlook may be less favourable. This is the case for most people whose heart failure is caused by a heart attack, high blood pressure or heart muscle disease. Even so, the situation is considerably better than it would have been just ten years ago, when studies suggested that the outlook was not good. Thanks to recent advances in medical care, many people with heart failure are surviving much longer. Treatment is much more effective if started early.

Although improved treatments can prolong the lives of many people with heart failure, what's equally important is that they can improve their quality of life too. As we saw on page 34, modern medicines can reduce, if not control, unpleasant and restricting symptoms such as breathlessness and enable people to continue enjoying life.

KEY POINTS

✓ It is fine to travel abroad as long as you take sensible precautions

✓ Make sure you know how to deal with dehydration (diarrhoea and vomiting)

✓ It is good to travel with a friend/relative who understands your condition in case of emergency

New frontiers

Advances in medicine are taking place all the time and, together with improved life expectancy and quality of life, the outlook for people who experience heart failure is steadily improving. This chapter gives an overview of the latest medicines and other treatments on the market.

DIAGNOSIS

Recent research suggests that a simple blood test may soon be available that can help doctors detect heart failure early and monitor its progress.

It is now recognised that heart attacks may put only part of the heart muscle to sleep rather than killing it outright. In these patients treatment with beta-blockers or re-establishing the blood supply to the heart by a coronary artery bypass or with an angioplasty (pages 45–6)

may restore function to the 'sleeping' or 'hibernating' heart muscle. Detection of this sort of problem requires sophisticated tests, usually a heart scan with an injection of a small amount of radioactivity or a special type of echocardiography (see page 29).

It is also clear that heart failure caused by small, stiff hearts is much more common than previously known. Doctors know less about this problem and how to treat it. It is not clear whether standard treatments for heart failure are effective for this problem.

NEW PILLS

Before new medications can become available for use, they all have to be shown to be of proven value and safety; this is achieved through clinical research trials, before their use is widely recommended. Most of the following are already available but not yet widely used for heart failure.

Cholesterol-lowering medicines

Examples of these medicines are bezafibrate (Bezalip), simvastatin (Zocor), pravastatin (Lipostat), atorvastatin, gemfibrozil (Lopid). High cholesterol predisposes to atheroma (see Heart attack, page 12) and medicines that reduce cholesterol have been shown to reduce the risk of heart attacks. The safety and efficacy of these medicines have never been properly tested in heart failure but many doctors feel that they should be helpful by reducing the risk of further heart damage.

Vasopeptidase, vasopressin and endothelin blockers

Many new compounds are being developed that block chemical messengers other than angiotensin (see ACE inhibitors, pages 34–5). Whether or not these will produce useful benefits for patients awaits further research.

NEW DEVICES

Telemonitoring

Careful supervision of patients with heart failure by a nurse or a doctor can improve how they feel, help them stay out of hospital, and live a longer and better life. Unfortunately, there are usually too many patients for the health service to cope. One way of helping doctors and nurses to keep a close eye on patients is to supply special devices to measure weight, blood pressure, and heart rate and rhythm, with the information sent automatically by radio signals and telephone lines to the doctor's health centre or the local hospital. This is called telemonitoring. This may give the doctor early warning of deterioration, allowing the doctor to give treatment to prevent a crisis and to keep the patient out of hospital.

NEW SURGERY

Transplanting animal hearts

If a human receives a live animal organ, the body's immune system rapidly rejects it. Genetically engineered pigs have been developed that have an immune system similar to that of humans. The first transplants of these genetically altered pig hearts should take place within the next few years. This strategy, if successful, could overcome the shortage of human hearts for transplantation.

Artificial hearts

Over the last few years mechanical hearts have been developed to take over the function of the failing heart temporarily in very sick patients in whom a heart for transplantation could not be found immediately. A small number of patients have now waited for 1–2 years for a transplant. Doctors are now considering whether a 'real heart' is required for these patients. However, mechanical hearts are very expensive. Clots forming inside the mechanical heart can be a problem, leading to complications such as stroke. Mechanical hearts are recommended mainly as a 'stop-gap' measure while awaiting transplantation and in a few other exceptional cases. However, new developments are making these sorts of devices cheaper, safer and more efficient.

KEY POINTS

✓ Advances in medicines are taking place all the time

✓ The outlook for people who experience heart failure is steadily improving

Useful addresses

British Heart Foundation
14 Fitzhardinge Street
London W1H 6DH
Tel: 020 7935 0185
Fax: 020 7486 5820
Helpline: 08450 708 070 (24 hours)
Website: www.bhf.org.uk

This charity funds vital research into heart disease, and life-saving equipment, rehabilitation centres and heart support groups. It also educates the public and the professionals. It depends on donations from the public for this work.

Cardiomyopathy Association
40 The Metro Centre
Tolpits Lane
Watford
Hertfordshire WD18 9SB
Freephone: 0800 0181 024
Tel: 01923 249977
Fax: 01923 249987
Email: cmaassoc@aol.com
Website: www.cardiomyopathy.org

Support organisation helping patients and medical professionals with information on hypertrophic, dilated and other forms of cardiomyopathy.

Diabetes UK
10 Parkway
London NW1 7AA
Careline: 020 7424 1030 (9am–5pm)
Tel: 020 7424 1000
Fax: 020 7424 1001
Email: info@diabetes.org.uk
Website: www.diabetes.org.uk

Supplies information on diabetes and its connection with heart disease.

Health Development Agency
7th Floor, Holborn Gate
330 High Holborn
London WC1V 7BA
Tel: 020 7430 0850
Fax: 020 7061 3390
Email: communications@hda-online.org.uk
Website: www.hda-online.org.uk

A special health authority, working to improve the health of people and communities in England, in particular to reduce health inequalities. In partnership with others, it gathers evidence of what works, advises on standards and develops the skills of all those working to improve people's health.

NHS Direct
Freephone: **0845 4647** (24 hours)

Trained operatives will assess symptoms and give advice on the level of care needed, as well as provide general information.

Lifesavers, The Royal Life Saving Society UK
River House, High Street
Broom
Warwickshire B50 4HN
Tel: 01789 773994
Fax: 01789 773995
Email: mail@rlss.org.uk
Website: www.lifesavers.org.uk

Runs life support courses throughout the UK.

St John Ambulance
27 St John's Lane
London EC1M 4BU
Tel: 020 7324 4000
Fax: 020 7324 4001
Website: www.sja.org.uk

Resuscitation Council (UK)
5th Floor, Tavistock House North
Tavistock Square
London WC1H 9HR
Tel: 020 7388 4678
Fax: 020 7383 0773
Email enquiries@resus.org.uk
Website: www.resus.org.uk

The Council facilitates the education of the public and professionals in effective resuscitation methods.

Smoking Quitlines
England: **0800 002200**
N. Ireland: **028 9066 3281**
Scotland (Smokeline): **0800 848484** (12 noon–midnight)
Wales: **0800 169 0 169**

THE INTERNET AS A SOURCE OF FURTHER INFORMATION

After reading this book, you may feel that you would like further information on the subject. One source is the internet and there are a great many websites with useful information about medical disorders, related charities and support groups. Some websites, however, have unhelpful and inaccurate information. Many are sponsored by commercial organisations or raise revenue by advertising, but nevertheless aim to provide impartial and trustworthy health information. Others may be reputable but you should be aware that they may be biased in their recommendations. Remember that treatment advertised on international websites may not be available in the UK.

Unless you know the address of the specific website that you want to visit (for example, familydoctor.co.uk), you may find the following guidelines helpful when searching the internet.

There are several different sorts of websites that you can use to look for information, the main ones being search engines, directories and portals.

Search engines and directories
There are many search engines and directories that all use different algorithms (procedures for computation) to return different results when you do a search. Search engines use computer programs called spiders, which crawl the web on a daily basis to search individual pages within a site and then queue them ready for listing in their database.

Directories, however, consider a site as a whole and use the description and information that was provided with the site when it was submitted to the directory to decide whether a site matches the searcher's needs. For both there is little or no selection in terms of quality of information, although engines and directories do try to

impose rules about decency and content. Popular search engines in the UK include:

> google.co.uk
> aol.co.uk
> msn.co.uk
> lycos.co.uk
> hotbot.co.uk
> overture.com
> ask.co.uk
> espotting.com
> looksmart.co.uk
> alltheweb.com
> uk.altavista.com

The two biggest directories are:

> yahoo.com
> dmoz.org

Portals
Portals are doorways to the internet that provide links to useful sites, news and other services, and may also provide search engine services (such as msn.co.uk). Many portals charge for putting their clients' sites high up in your list of search results. The quality of the websites listed depends on the selection criteria used in compiling the portal, although portals focused on a specific group, such as medical information portals, may have more rigorous inclusion criteria than other searchable websites. Examples of medical portals can be found at:

nhsdirect.nhs.uk
patient.co.uk

Links to many British medical charities will be found at the Association of Medical Research Charities (www.amrc.org.uk) and Charity Choice (www.charitychoice.co.uk).

Search phrases

Be specific when entering a search phrase. Searching for information on 'cancer' could give astrological information as well as medical: 'lung cancer' would be a better choice. Either use the engine's advanced search feature and ask for the exact phrase, or put the phrase in quotes – 'lung cancer' – as this will link the words. Adding 'uk' to your search phrase will bring up mainly British websites, so a good search would be 'lung cancer' uk (don't include uk within the quotes).

Always remember that the internet is international and unregulated. Although it holds a wealth of invaluable information, individual websites may be biased, out of date or just plain wrong. Family Doctor Publications accepts no responsibility for the content of links published in their series.

Index

ACE inhibitors **4, 34–5, 42–3, 52, 55, 61, 62**
 – and water tablets **37**
adrenaline blocking **38**
age as risk factor **3, 12**
alcohol, as risk factor **3, 18, 20, 51, 61**
 – warfarin and **43**
aldosterone **38**
alpha-blockers **42–3**
amiodarone **41, 61, 62**
amlodipine **42**
anaemia, as risk factor **20**
 – testing for **27**
aneurysmectomy **46**
angina **21**
 – treatment **40**
angiograms **31**
angioplasty **45–6**
angiotensin **34**
angiotensin II blockers **35–6, 42–3**
ankles, checking **26**
 – swollen **2, 3, 4, 10, 23, 24**
 – treatment **36**
anticoagulants **42–3**
antihistamine patches **60**
antiplatelets **42–3**
aorta **8**
aortic valve **9**
 – damage **17**
arteries, heart **5, 8**
 – damage **15–16**
 – surgery **45–6**
 – tests **31**
artery wall, damaged **15**
 – normal **15**
artificial hearts **69–70**

aspirin **40**
asthma, beta-blockers and **38**
atheroma **12, 13**
atorvastatin **69**
atria **7, 8, 9**
atrial fibrillation **7, 16–17, 20, 39**
 – treatment **33, 36**
atrial systole **7**
atrioventricular node **9**

beta-blockers **38–9, 42–3, 52**
bezafibrate **69**
bicycle test **30**
bisoprolol **38, 42–3**
blood clots **12, 16, 17**
 – formation **43**
 – treatment **36, 40, 43**
blood, deoxygenated **9**
 – oxygenated **5, 9**
 – supplying nutrients and oxygen **10**
 – tests **27, 37**
 – thinning **17, 40, 43**
 – volume **7**
blood flow **9**
 – around body **6**
 – in heart **5**
blood pressure, checking **26**
 – normal **14**
 – test **14, 15**
 – see also high blood pressure
blood vessels, dilation **34**
 – leaking fluid **24**
 – narrowed, surgery **44–5**
brain, blood clots in **17**
breathlessness **2, 3, 4, 10, 22–4, 38, 53**

breathlessness (contd)
- from amiodarone **43**
- gradual **55**
- improvements **52**
- sudden **54**
- treatment **36**
British Heart Foundation **60, 71**

calcification of tissues **19**
calcium channel blockers **41, 42–3, 44, 54**
capillaries, leaking **10**
car travel **60**
cardiac glycosides **41–2**
cardiomyopathy **18, 20**
- dilated **5**
Cardiomyopathy Association **71**
cardiovascular system **5**
cardioversion **33, 44**
carvedilol **38, 42–3**
causes of heart failure **12–21**
chart for progress monitoring **57–8**
chemical messengers and heart failure **10**
chest, pain **54**
- X-ray **27**
children and heart failure **3**
cholesterol, high, and high blood pressure **15**
- as risk factor **3**
cholesterol-lowering medicine **69**
circulatory system **5–7**
clot-busting medicine **14**
confusion **4**
congenital heart defect **18, 19**
coronary arteries **8, 12, 13**
- bypass graft **45**
- disease **2, 49**
- infarction **12**
- tests **31**
coughing **2**
- from treatment **35**

defibrillators, implantable **47**
dehydration while travelling **61**
diabetes, beta-blockers and **38**
- as risk factor **3**
Diabetes UK **71**
diagnosing heart failure **22–31**
- advances **68**
diarrhoea, water tablets and **37, 62**
diastole **7**

diastolic blood pressure **14**
diet **50–1, 57**
- causing anaemia **20**
digoxin **39**
diuretics *see* water tablets
dizziness **37, 38**
- from treatment **35, 37, 55**
doctor–patient relationship **56**

echocardiography **29, 66**
electric shock treatment **33, 44**
electrocardiogram (ECG) **28**
emergencies **63**
endocarditis **18, 19**
endothelin blockers **69**
enlarged heart **27**
exercise **51, 52, 57**
- and heart beat **7**
- test 30

family concern **62–3**
fatigue *see* tiredness
fats in diet **51**
fatty deposits **12**
fibre in diet **51**
floppy valves **19**
fluid, intake on holiday **62**
- retention **10, 21, 22–4, 27, 44, 51, 53, 54–5**
- treatment **36**
flying **60–2**
frequently asked questions on heart failure **63**
friends' concern **62–3**
frusemide **38**

gangrene **17**
gemfibrozil **69**
generic names **34**
genetics, anaemia **20**
- heart disease **18**
gout **37**
great vein **8**
GTN *see* nitrates

haemoglobin **20**
Health Development Agency **71**
heart **8–9**
- artificial **69–70**
- baggy **20**
- enlargement **27**
- how it works **5–11**

– normal **15**
– protection **36**
– pumping cycle **7**
– scan **30, 68**
– sounds, checking **26**
heart attack, as risk factor **12–14**
– effects **1, 3 , 45**
heart beat, abnormalities treatment **43**
– beta-blockers and **38**
– control **39**
– irregularity **7**
– control **39, 44**
– testing **28**
heart disease vs heart failure **21**
heart failure, what is it? **1–2**
heart muscle **5, 9**
– death **3, 13, 14**
– disease **18, 20**
– sleeping **45, 68**
– testing **29**
– thickening **15**
heart transplants, animal **69**
heart valves *see* valves *and specific valves*
hibernating heart **45, 68**
high altitude and heart failure **60**
high blood pressure **4**
– as risk factor **2, 3, 14–16, 19**
– treatment **35, 38, 41, 42–3, 44**
holidays **60–2**
hormones and heart failure **10**
hypertension, essential **15**
– *see mainly* high blood pressure
hypertrophic cardiomyopathy **20**

ibuprofen interactions **53–4**
immune suppression after transplants **47**
immune system disorders **18**
immunisations **60**
infections of heart valve **19**
insurance **60**
ischaemic disease **19**

jaundice from amiodarone **41**

kidney, as risk factor **21**
– diuretics and **36**
– passing urine **24, 37**
– problems **10**
– ACE inhibitors and **35**

– and digoxin **39**
– and high blood pressure **15**
– testing for **27**
– salt and water retention **34**

leg, blood clots in **17, 24**
– swelling **24**
Lifesavers **72**
lifestyle changes **49–53**
liver, amiodarone and **41**
lung, amiodarone and **41**
– damage from smoking **49**
– disease **27**
– fluid-filled **10, 23, 24, 27**

medication **33–4**
– how they are given **40**
– interactions **53–4**
– new **68–9**
– noting side effects **52, 55**
– timing **52**
– trade names **33–4**
menstrual bleeding causing anaemia **20**
metoprolol **38, 42–3**
mitral valve **9**
– damage **17**
mixed valve disease **18**
monitoring progress **52–4, 57–8**
muscle *see* heart muscle
muscular dystrophy as risk factor **3**
myocardial infarction **12**

nausea and vomiting, digoxin and **39**
neck, checking **26**
NHS Direct **72**
nitrates **39–40, 42–3, 54**
nutrient supply **10**
– poor **23**

obesity and high blood pressure **15**
outlook for heart failure **66**
oxygen, delivery problems **20**
– levels in smokers **49**
– supply **10**
– poor **23**

pacemakers **46–7**
palpitations **7**
paralysis in limbs **17**
physical examination **25, 26**

pig heart transplants **69**
plaques **12, 13**
platelets in blood **40**
potassium chloride in diet **50**
potassium loss **37–8**
pravastatin **69**
pregnancy as risk factor **3**
progress checking **52–4, 58–9**
proprietary names *see* trade names
prostate gland, enlarged **24**
– problems **37**
pulmonary artery **8**
pulmonary valve **9**
pulse checking **26**
pulses in diet **51**
pump efficiency **5**

regurgitation **17, 19**
relaxation classes **57**
Resuscitation Council **72**
resuscitation technique **63, 64**
rheumatic fever **17–18, 19**
risk factors for heart attack **3, 12, 63, 66**

salt, in diet **50**
– high, and high blood pressure **15**
– intake on holiday **62**
– retention **44**
saturated fats in diet **51**
save-a-life course **63**
scans **30, 69**
scar tissue following heart attack **5, 13, 14**
– surgery for **46**
scientific names for medicines **34**
sea sickness **60**
sea travel **60**
self-help treatment **49–55**
self-monitoring chart **58–9**
sex life **57**
shortness of breath *see* breathlessness
side effects, noting **52, 55**
simvastin **69**
sinoatrial node **9**
sleep position, easing breathlessness **22**
– problems **2**
Smoking Quitlines **72**
smoking risks **3, 49–50, 57**

sodium chloride in diet **50**
sodium cromoglycate for cough **35**
sphygmomanometer **14**
spironolactone **38, 42–3**
St John Ambulance **72**
stenosis **17, 19**
stress **57**
– and travel **60–1**
stroke **16, 17, 43**
sunlight sensitivity **41, 61, 62**
surgery for heart failure **44–5**
swelling **10, 23**
– treatment **36**
symptoms of heart failure **2, 3, 22–5, 53–5, 63**
systolic blood pressure **14**

telemonitoring **69**
tests for heart failure **25–31**
thrombosis **12**
thyroid gland, overactivity **43**
– problems as risk factor **20–1**
thyroid hormone levels, testing for **27**
tiredness **2, 3, 4, 10, 23, 24, 38**
trade names for medicines **33–4**
train travel **60**
transport problems **60**
travel **60–2**
treadmill test **30**
treatment for heart failure **33–48**
– self-help **49–55**
tricuspid valve **9**
tummy upsets **61, 62**

uric acid formation **37**
urine, passing **24, 37, 38**
– retention **37**

valves, causes of disease **19**
– control of heart **5, 7**
– disorders **3, 17–18, 19**
– floppy **19**
– leaking **14, 17, 18**
– narrowing **17, 18**
– normal **18**
– regurgitation **17, 19**
– replacement **3, 44**
– surgery for **44**
– testing **29, 31**
vasopeptidase **69**
vasopressin **69**

veins, blood clots in **25**
 – distended **26**
ventricles **7, 9**
ventricular systole **7**
vomiting, water tablets and **62**

warfarin **40–1, 42**
 – and aspirin **40, 43**
 – and cardioversion **44**
waste products accumulation in
      tissues **23**
water tablets **1, 3, 36–8, 42–3, 52**
 – and ACE inhibitors **35**

 – on holiday **62**
weighing scales **53, 61, 62**
weight, fluctuations **36–7, 53, 61,
      62**
 – gain **53, 54–5**
   – from fluid retention **21**
 – loss **2, 43, 51**
   – dieting for **57**
weights, lifting **52**
wheezing **2**
who gets heart failure? **3**

X-rays **27**